In Loving Memory of Jeffrey H. Bower

Dedication

I dedicate this story to my wonderful, loving mother, Brendamae, who watched me suffer for a long time. Thanks Mom for never giving up on me. I also dedicated this story to my brother Justin, who kept loyal to me while I was in dire need of support. I want to thank you both for inspiring me to write my story. I love both of you very much. I also dedicate this story to Doctor Anne Tapley, whose inspiration helped me to speak of my trauma and hurt through my writing. I want to thank all of you for your support and advice that was very much needed. I also wish to thank my younger siblings. My goal is to one day have my story become a major motion picture.

Written by A E Bower
Autism- The Fight Inside

Editor: Austin E. Bower

Disclaimer

In my true life story: *Autism- The Fight Inside*, the names have been altered to protect the people who were really involved, for legal reasons of course. All the characters are real, and all the places are real. My story can be fact checked to prove just how real it is. If any names occur that are in my book, it is a pure coincidence, and I ensure you I altered the names. Also I am well aware of the Son of Sam law in the United States. This story is not about the robbery. This story is about the crime of our government failing me in the system while having a developmental disability and being sentenced to prison. My story reflects the lost boy who aged in the system. I address how the system failed me and neglected to see my disability by sending me to prison. It is my freedom of speech to tell my story of brokenness within my heart and within the system. Any royalties I receive I deserve for the simple fact that the story is not about the robbery. It is the story about how I was robbed. Also a non-fiction story is defined as having real events in the story take place. The names of people being altered still meet the qualifications of a non-fiction story. You can even look on the world wide web to check the definition yourselves.

Chapter 1 No Friend of Mine

One of the main characteristic's in autism is the inability to not trust some one. Meaning those with autism usually trust more than they should.

A*ugust 3th, 2009* was dark, and the moon was the only light shining in the night. Few people were out moving around in Lincoln, Nebraska. The air was moist, and families were off to bed. There were a few souls up, and they were only looking for trouble. Among those few were Hawkboy and myself. Hawkboy was a Native American, and his eyes were beady and brown. He was short with a dark complexion. He had tattoos covering his chest as he walked with his shirt off under the moon. I was walking alongside Hawkboy, and I was taller than him by a few inches. I was white with brown hair and green eyes. I had a few tattoos myself, one of which was on my back. *California* in Old English it read, and the tattoo was shoulder blade to shoulder blade.

"Austin, are you ready to party?" Hawkboy was asking me as he swayed back and forth.

"There's going to be a lot of girls there," Hawkboy said.

"Plus there will be a lot to drink too."

"I could use a drink," I said.

We continued walking down downtown Lincoln.

"So where is this party at?"

"Don't worry, we are almost there," he said.

"Are we going to take some girls back to my place?"

"Ya, we can do that," Hawkboy said.

We both walked down 19th and J Street side by side. The neighborhood had old, worn-down buildings, and the streets were quiet. I began to have a bad feeling in my gut about where Hawkboy was taking me. I thought it was odd that Hawkboy wasn't giving me any details as to where we were going.

"Where are we going, Hawkboy?"

"Don't worry about it. I said I was taking you to a party," Hawkboy said.

I tried not to read too much into it. I figured if Hawkboy was lying to me he would say so. I saw a man riding his bicycle, and Hawkboy began to chase after him. The man slowed down only for a moment, and then Hawkboy hit the man in the back of the head. The man fell to the ground, and he didn't look so good. The man tried to pick himself up, but Hawkboy stomped his head into the pavement. I noticed the man wasn't moving, and I began to walk away. I saw a flight of stairs, and I hid under the metal steps. I was very afraid of Hawkboy, and I noticed something in him had switched. Whatever it was, it was evil. I was crouched under a flight of stairs, and Hawkboy could see me.

"Hey, let's go," Hawkboy said.

I was frozen, and I didn't want to move. Hawkboy came walking in my direction, and I had a horrible feeling in my stomach.

"I said let's go, Austin," he said.

Hawkboy waited a few minutes, and I soon rejoined him. Hawkboy and I were on the sidewalk near a broken fence. We continued to head east. The streets were littered with cars of all different sizes and colors. Hawkboy led me to an apartment complex. The complex was dark red, and Hawkboy and I were on 18th and G Street. I saw another apartment with its lights on, so I ran to the front entrance. I opened the door, and I saw a phone. I grabbed the phone, and the phone led me to an operator. I looked up in the small hallway and I noticed a camera. The camera was looking right at me.

"Hello," I said.

"Please let me in!"

The operator didn't know me, but they buzzed me in anyway. The door to the complex opened, and I

7

walked in. I tried to shut the door behind me, but Hawkboy was too quick for me.

"What are you doing?"

"Nothing," I said.

The fear was seen in my eyes.

"Let's go," he said.

I was too afraid to say no, and I didn't want to be attacked. As Hawkboy and I exited the complex, he grabbed the camera and tore it down. From there Hawkboy led me to 17th and G Street. We were both standing outside of a brick apartment complex.

"Okay, we're here," Hawkboy said.

"So let's go in then," I said.

"Not so fast," Hawkboy said.

"We're not here to party, Austin."

"We're here to rob this guy," he said.

"Whoa, hold on," I said.

"You never said anything about a robbery."

"Austin, chill little homie. It will be all right," Hawkboy said.

"Look, man," I said, "I came here to party. I didn't come here to rob some guy."

"Austin, he is a drug dealer. If we rob him, he won't call the cops," he explained.

8

"No, I can't do this," I replied.

"Motherfucker, you're gonna help me whether you want to or not!"

"Loyalty," he said.

"Man, this isn't a good idea," I whispered.

I had my head down, and I was afraid to look Hawkboy in his eyes.

"If you're not in here in five seconds," Hawkboy threatened, "I will find you, and I will kick your ass my damn self!"

"Now get your fucking ass up here," he said.

Hawkboy was whispering aggressively.

"Okay, fine," I said.

The door was at the top of the steps, and Hawkboy and I climbed the steps until we reached the second floor. The door was red, and it had the number eight. Hawkboy approached the door and looked around briefly. Then Hawkboy took his leg, and thrust his body into the door, and the door swung wide open.

"Crack, bang, slam!" The door rang out in my ears.

The sound of wood and metal breaking caused me to freeze. I stood there as Hawkboy rushed into the apartment. The door hung on a hinge, and the door was falling apart. For a little guy Hawkboy had some power behind him.

"Where's the fucking money? Give me the fucking money!"

Hawkboy was hitting a man over and over again.

"Give me the fucking money," he said again.

I walked into the apartment, and there was a man laying on the sofa in the living room. The living room was littered with trash and cups along with bowls and bags of dog food. A small dog was barking over and over again. The dog was tiny and looked like the size of a junior football. I walked closer to the action, and I had no idea what to do. I was frozen in time. There was blood everywhere, and Hawkboy had blood all over his shirt. The man looked old. He had to be in his fifties, and he was Mexican.

"Austin, help me," Hawkboy said.

I ignored his command, and I threw no punches. I decided to move toward the living room near the front door. As I did, the fight was brought out into the living room. Hawkboy was hitting the man over and over again.

"Hawkboy, get off me!"

Holy shit, this guy knows him, I thought. I picked Hawkboy up off of the ground and body slammed him into a bike rack that was in the corner of the living room. Hawkboy and the old man fell together. As Hawkboy tried to get up, he lost his shoe in the process. Hawkboy ran out the door, and I followed close behind. We were both on foot now, and Hawkboy was limping and needed another shoe. We were outside and running behind the apartment complex. Street lights were glowing, and the pavement was glistening. As we ran it sounded like cards shuffling due to our jeans making friction.

"Austin, why would you do that?"

"I don't know, I just reacted," I said.

"Fuck, Austin," Hawkboy said.

"Fuck!"

We both ran east through backyards, climbing fences to homes that didn't belong to us. At one point we were behind some bushes that faced the street. I saw a police cruiser posted up just sitting there. Hawkboy tried to make a move, but I stopped him.

"What, are you crazy?"

"There's a cop right there," I said.

I was whispering to keep a low profile. The officer just sat there, and we both waited until he left. Eventually he did, and we were back on foot again. Hawkboy walked up to a family's house and saw shoes lined up on the front porch. Hawkboy grabbed a shoe and began to put it on his shoeless foot. It didn't fit him, but it was the only one that seemed close to his size. Hawkboy and I continued to run several more blocks. We finally returned to my apartment. I lived at 456 South 26th Street. We were looking around to be sure the police didn't follow us. I had a key to my apartment, but I was shaking too much to unlock the door. Finally I got the door open, and Hawkboy went straight to the sofa to lay down.

"Look, I have one hundred and three dollars," Hawkboy said.

"That was from the robbery?"

"Yep," he said.

"What if this guy calls the cops?"

"He won't, he's a drug dealer," Hawkboy said.

"I don't know, man, you just robbed the guy. Plus you beat him up pretty bad," I said.

My living room had a yellow sofa and a brown carpet. I had a bathroom near my bedroom, and my bedroom had a mattress. My clothing was scattered everywhere, and my dishes were unfinished. I had a coffee table in front of my yellow sofa. On my coffee table was a Bible and a few other books. Hawkboy took the one hundred and three dollars and put it inside my Bible.

"No, you can't put that money in there," I said.

"Why not? It's only a Bible."

"Ya, well it's my Bible," I said.

"Okay," he replied.

12

Hawkboy kept the stolen money in my Bible with no regard to what I said. Thankfully the police hadn't shown up at my house, and it was getting late. So I decided to lay down. I went to my mattress, and I laid down until I fell asleep.

The next morning after the robbery, Hawkboy was awake on my sofa. I went into the kitchen to get some food, and I noticed my milk was gone. I knew that I didn't drink it. I figured it was Hawkboy, because he was the only one in my house.

"Hey, Austin," Hawkboy said.

"What?"

"Monia is coming over to spend some time with us," he said.

Hawkboy had a lady friend named Monia. She was Mexican and had long black hair. Her skin was dark brown, and she had brown eyes. Hawkboy was looking at his phone.

"Okay," I said.

"What time will she be here?"

"She didn't say, but she's bringing her van," he said.

Her mini van was a green 1994 Mercury.

"Okay," I said.

I peeked my head into the living room from where I was standing in the kitchen.

"Hey, what happened to all my milk?"

"I drank it," he replied.

"Okay.... next time let me know before you do," I said.

"Why?"

"Because now I have nothing to eat for breakfast," I said.

"You'll be all right, just chill, little homie."

I went the entire morning without having any food, and I felt like I needed something to eat. I went to the cabinet to get my medication, and I saw that my bottle was empty. I was bothered by this.

"Hawkboy!"

It was visible that I was upset.

"What?"

"Where is my medication?"

"Oh, those belonged to you?"

"Ya man, my name's right on bottle," I said.

"I sold them last night," he said.

"What?"

I could feel an argument rising.

"To who?"

"Don't worry about it," he said.

14

"Don't worry about it? I needed those," I fumed.

"You'll be all right."

"Fuck, Hawkboy," I said.

"Just chill out and relax," he said.

Hawkboy sat up and I sat next to him on the sofa. We waited until Monia showed up. In the meantime, Hawkboy decided to call his drug dealer to see what was going on. I watched as he dialed the number on his cell phone.

"Chiko," Hawkboy said.

"What's up?"

He was on speakerphone so I could hear his voice.

"This is Hawkboy," he said.

"I know who this is," Chiko said.

"Did you call the police?"

"Ya, I called the cops," Chiko said.

"No, you didn't," Hawkboy said.

"Yes, I did," Chiko said.

"Why would you do that?"

"Because you robbed me," Chiko said. "I hope you get locked up too, motherfucker."

"Fuck you, punk!"

Then Hawkboy ended the phone call.

15

"Fuck, he called the cops," Hawkboy said.

Hawkboy was starring at his cell phone.

"Ya, he did," I said. "We're fucked."

"Don't think like that," Hawkboy said.

"How am I supposed to think? You robbed the guy," I said.

"It will be all right," Hawkboy assured me.

"You need to leave."

"I'm not going anywhere," Hawkboy said.

"You need to leave now!"

"Are you trying to fight me, Austin?"

"No. But you need to leave," I stated.

"I'm staying right here," he said.

I was defeated, and I didn't know what to do. I decided to take a seat. I sat on the sofa, hungry and without my medication. I knew this was wrong, and I knew I was in trouble.

Knock, knock, knock. Someone knocked at the door.

It had to be Monia.

I went to open the door, and Monia walked in, carrying her purse on her shoulder. I was relieved to know she wasn't the police.

"Hey Hawkboy, how are you?" Monia asked while

smiling at Hawkboy, and he gave her a hug.

"Good....I'm good," he said.

"You got the weed?"

"Ya, right here," Monia said.

She dug in her purse and pulled out a bag of a green. Monia had her hair in a bun, and she wore red sweatpants and a black t-shirt.

"Let's smoke it up," Monia said.

Monia pulled out a pipe and a liter, and I felt uncomfortable.

"Hawkboy, I think I'm gonna leave," I said.

"No, stay," he said.

"I don't know, man."

"Seriously, stay and smoke some bud with us," he said.

"I'm gonna go," I replied.

"Okay, be that way," Hawkboy said.

I decided to leave, and I walked around the neighborhood. I looked at the trees, and I watched the birds in the air. The sun was beginning to fall as the moon took over, as if the moon and sun had a relationship with one another, dancing in a beautiful gleaming light while taking turns with their shifts. Guarding the hearts of humanity by being loyal to mankind. I soon returned home hoping that Hawkboy would be gone. On my arrival my hopes were dismissed. I walked into my apartment, and I sat on the floor. The sofa was controlled by Hawkboy and Monia.

"I have a friend who's coming over," Monia said.

"That's cool," Hawkboy said.

Hawkboy answered to her every word, as if they had a solid relationship. However I knew what they had was superficial.

The day went by with nothing productive. Meaningless conversation happened, and the day faded into the night. Monia's friend never came over, and Monia decided to stay the night. We listened to the radio all throughout the night. I had no medication to take, and I could sense myself being off balance. I didn't own a television, so I decided to lay down. I went to lay down, and I couldn't fall asleep. My eyes just wouldn't shut, and I knew it was because I needed my medication. So I laid there for the entire night and decided to do nothing. The hours seemed to drag on, and I started to worry about the police arresting me for a robbery that I didn't even do. I just happened to be with this crook. There was something about him that was demonic. I believed there was something about him that was just plain evil, and he was in my house. I laid on my mattress all night, thinking of ways to get away from this guy. The next day presented itself, and I felt like I had to go. I felt too unsafe to stay in my own apartment. I needed a car if I wanted to get out quickly. I needed my medications too. I just had to convince Monia to let me borrow her van. She was just waking up, and so was Hawkboy. Monia went into the bathroom, and I waited until she came out. As Monia came out into the living room, I approached her.

"Monia, can I borrow your van?"

"For what?"

She wasn't expecting for me to ask such a question.

Her hair was messy, and she was playing with it.

"To get us some food," I said.

"I don't know..."

She questioned my intentions, but I couldn't tell her I wasn't coming back.

"Please? I will be right back," I said.

I lied directly to her face.

"I'm going to drive to the supermarket."

"And buy what?"

"Food," I said.

The question was stupid because I just told her that I wanted to buy food.

Hawkboy came into the living room from the bathroom.

"What's going on?"

"Austin wants to drive to the supermarket," Monia said.

"Let him," he said.

"Okay," Monia replied.

After Hawkboy said it was okay, she to listened to that. Either way I wasn't coming back, and I knew it too. I headed out the door, and I noticed the sky was blue. I also noticed a police cruiser seated near my driveway. I walked into the grass and down the curb where the van was parked. My apartment sat on a hill. The van was green, and one of the tires looked to be going flat. I unlocked the driver's side door, and I sat in the driver's seat. I put the key into the ignition, and I began to pull off. I saw the police cruiser tailing me in my rear view mirror. I took the long way to the exit from my apartment complex, which was by driving behind the building. I did this to beat the officer. I began to drive eastbound, and I took J Street. I also noticed there were a lot of cars in traffic. I went past the lights on 27th and J, and I continued to drive. I made it to 29th and J before the officer turned their lights on. The lights signaled blue and red, but I kept driving until I reached 30th and J. I eventually made a complete stop. The officer got out of the vehicle, and I noticed the officer was a woman. She approached the van and began to speak to me.

20

"License and registration?"

I looked at her closely. She was wearing sunglasses and her uniform was black and blue. What I noticed most was her gun. I handed her my license through the window, and she walked back to her vehicle. Her lights were still flashing. She was in her car for about two minutes. When she walked back, it didn't look like she had good news to give me.

"Do you have registration for this vehicle?"

"I'm borrowing it," I said.

"From who?"

"Monia Shell," I said.

"Well, you have a warrant out for your arrest," she said, "so I need you to step out of the vehicle."

"No, I'm not going anywhere with you," I said.

"Sir, please step out of the van."

"No," I said.

"Sir, please step out of the vehicle."

"No, go fuck yourself," I said.

I started the ignition switch to the van, and I took off in a hurry. I saw her run back to her police car in my rear view mirror. I drove at the speed of twenty miles per hour, picking up more speed. I was approaching a stoplight, but I kept driving anyways. The police cruiser was gaining on me, and I needed to get away.

I picked up speed, going sixty miles per hour in a twenty-five mile per hour zone. I drove past parked cars and people walking. I was picking up more speed, and I had no intent to slow down. I reached ninety miles per hour in a twenty-five per hour zone. I was coming up to an intersection that wouldn't let me travel straight through. I slowed down, quickly pumping my breaks, and I turned left at the intersection. The tires were skidding as I made my full turn. I made the turn successfully, but I had another turn to make. This time on the right, and the turn was sharper than the last. Cars were parked all along the intersection that I was turning into. The turn was so sharp that I blew the right tire to the van. The van began to hump up and down. I soon realized I wouldn't make it far. So I decided to jump out and run on foot. I jumped out of the van as it was slowing down, and I ran up a hill on 42th and N Street. I continued to run, and as I did I was being chased. I ran behind a few businesses and houses, and I made my way to 44th and O Street. I was nearing a gas station. I kept running uphill, and then I was stopped by surrounding police officers. I noticed that I had nowhere else to go, and nowhere else to turn. The police surrounded me and placed me in handcuffs. I was already on the ground when they cuffed me. I knew it was over, and they knew it too.

Chapter 2 Police

Autism is a developmental disability however in some cases autism is not recognized by the human eye. Due to the fact that there are those who have less symtoms with the diagnosis, yet they are still very disabled.

I was brought into a small room in handcuffs, and the officer led me to a chair. I was seated in a plastic chair behind a table. The officer came in the room with a photo of Hawkboy and me outside of an apartment complex near where the robbery took place. The police officer removed my handcuffs.

"Is this you?"

The officer placed the photo on the table.

"No," I said.

"Well it looks like you," he said.

The officer was wearing a blue uniform, and he had a gun on his waistband. He had a short haircut, and it looked military. He had brown skin and brown eyes.

"It's not me," I said. "Honest."

"Well, we know it's you," he said.

"Okay, it's me, but that photo doesn't tell the whole

story," I said.

"Did you rob Chiko Herendez?"

"Who?"

"Chiko," he said.

"No, I didn't rob anyone," I said. "I was there, but I didn't rob anyone."

"You were there, but you didn't rob anyone?"

The officer wasn't convinced, and he was being sarcastic.

"No, honest, I didn't rob anyone," I said.

"But you were there?"

"Ya, I was there," I said.

"Okay, you're under arrest for the robbery of Chiko Herendez," he announced. "You have the right to remain silent."

"Wow, wow, hold on," I said.

"You have the right to an attorney. And if you can't afford one we will appoint one to you."

After I was read my Miranda rights, I was placed back in handcuffs, and I was led out of the small room. I was led from the interrogation unit to the county jail, which was next door. I was escorted by a male police officer. We both entered a room that had little cabinets. The officer took one of his keys, and he opened the cabinet. He placed his weapon into the

24

small cabinet, and then he locked it. The cabinet was metal and thick. The officer led me into an elevator, and the elevator led me to booking. We arrived at the top of the unit, and we were in front of a large, bulky door. The door was controlled by the guards who were inside. The guards cleared the door, and I was led in by the officer.

"I have Austin Bower here," Gibble said. "He is here on robbery two."

"Okay, stand over here, Bower," Dumble said.

Dumble was female, and she had a short haircut. I stood where she instructed me to, and a male guard came to pat me down.

"Take off your shoes," he said.

"Okay."

I took my shoes off one by one.

"Okay, place your hands on the counter," he instructed.

The counter was long and wide. There were computers behind the counter. I could also see files and paperwork organized in piles.

"Come with me," he said, "so I can strip search you."

The guard was old and white. He had white hair and a long nose. He led me into a hallway that led me into a strip out room. As I walked the hallway, I saw cells arranged in sections. I saw a few inmates in these cells. They appeared to be single cells, and the cells had large windows. The guard took me to the cell he wanted me in, and he opened the door.

"Step in," he said.

I did as he asked.

"Take off your clothes," he said.

"What?"

"Take off your clothes," he repeated.

"No."

He looked me up and down.

"Are we going to have a problem?"

"No," I said.

"Then take off your clothing," he insisted.

I began to take my clothes off. I started with my shirt and then went to my pants.

"The boxers too," he said.

I took my boxers off as he instructed.

"Now lift up your heels," he said.

I lifted my heels as he instructed.

"Now turn around," he said. "Now lift up your balls."

"What?"

"God dammit, lift up your balls," he said.

"Okay," I reluctantly agreed.

"Now turn around," he said.

I did everything he asked of me.

"Now bend over and spread your ass cheeks," he said.

"What?"

It was evident I didn't want to do this.

"Man, you're taking this too far," I said.

"Do it right now," he said.

I bent over and spread my cheeks.

"Now cough," he said.

I coughed as he instructed.

"Okay, pick up your shit and get dressed," he said.

I picked my clothing up, and I got dressed. He led me down the hallway and into a cell that was larger than the other ones. He opened the door, and I was housed with three other inmates. The guards were passing out lunch trays, and I was given stale hot dogs.

"Hey, can I make a phone call?"

"No," the guard said.

"Why not? I need to make my call," I said.

"You need to wait," he said.

"No, I want to make my phone call," I persisted.

"Well, you're not gonna," he said.

The guard had a bald head and a large upper body.

"Please, I really need to make my call," I said.

"Go back in your cell and shut up," he growled.

"Sir, I'm already in my cell," I said, "so how can I go back into my cell, sir?"

"We have a wise guy here. You know what? You just lost your phone privileges."

"What the fuck? Come on, man, please let me make my phone call," I said.

I began to reason with him.

"I want my phone call."

"You should of thought about that before you broke the law," he said.

"What the fuck? Sir, please can you let me use the phone?"

"No," he said.

I went towards the back of the cell, and I sat down on the floor. The cell had a toilet with nasty toilet water in it. I could tell the toilet hadn't been cleaned for months. There was no toilet paper either, and the ground was dirty and unkempt. The bench was taken, so I had nowhere else to sit. I sat on the floor, and I waited until the guards decided to move me.

"Bower, get up," the guard said.

He was a male guard, and he was short and skinny.

"We're moving you to general population," he said.

He opened the door and escorted me to the front desk.

"What are your sizes?"

"Extra large shirt and extra large pants," I said.

"Okay. Here, come with me. Take this towel and wash cloth. And this shampoo too."

"Okay," I said.

He led me to the back of the hallway.

"Here is the shower." He unlocked the door and moved to the side.

"Step in," he said.

It seemed like he paused every time he spoke a word.

"Take your shower."

I stepped in and he locked the door behind me. The shower had a button that made the water run. The water was cold, and the faucet had low water pressure. I took my shower, and I used the shampoo. The shampoo was blue and had a weird texture to it. I had no shower shoes on my feet, and that bothered me. I knew without shower shoes I would get athlete's foot. After my shower I dried off and I dressed myself.

"Hey I'm done," I said.

I pounded on the door a few times, and no one answered. I soon realized that they came when they wanted to. I was now on their watch, and I was no longer on my watch. The guard eventually returned, and he escorted me back to the front desk, and from there he had me wait. He finished up his paperwork. Then the guard gave me a blue bucket for my property. I watched him as he placed clothing into the property bucket. He also put in a drinking cup and a county jail handbook. The county jail handbook was orange and had the Nebraska seal on the front of it.

"Your escort is on the way, Bower," he said.

"Okay."

I waited another ten minutes, and my escort finally showed up. She was black with dreadlocks for her hair.

"Is he all set?" Her voice had a low tone to it.

"Ya, he's good to go," he said.

The guard seemed to not even care.

"Okay, come with me," she said.

I followed the guard through the hall while I carried my blue bucket. She escorted me through three doors on the way. I soon arrived to general population, and I saw nearly thirty inmates on the unit. Some inmates were writing letters, and a few others were on the phone. There were inmates seated at the tables too, and they looked to be separated by race. I had my bucket in my hands.

"Okay, Bower, you're in cell nineteen," she said.

She opened the door and left all at the same time, leaving me alone on the unit with my new fellow inmates. As I entered the unit, there were five blacks seated at the far right table. There were four whites seated at the far left table. There were two Mexicans seated right in front of me, near the door. Then there were two Native's seated across from the Mexicans. I began to walk my belongings to my cell, and the guard didn't open my cell door. So I decided to place my belongings in front of my cell door. I began to walk near the Native Americans, and they were both staring at me closely. I sat down near the book cart, and I began to look at the books. All of a sudden the guard came on to the unit. She was white with brown hair, and she was tall too.

"Open gym! Who wants to go to open gym?"

I really wanted to play basketball, so I lined up for gym. The blacks didn't line up, and neither did the Mexicans, but the whites and Natives did. There were four whites and two Natives with me in line, making a total of seven altogether.

"Let's go," she said.

I looked at the guard's name tag up close as we were

31

walking, and it read *Billingsly*. I could feel a strange vibe coming from the Natives and the whites. It was almost like they were at war with each other. The guard led me and the other inmates through two doors. She led us through the hallway that led to the gym. She unlocked the door to the gym and let us inside. I was the first one in, and the rest followed behind.

"Have fun," she said.

After that Billingsly shut the door behind her. I walked over to grab a basketball, and one of the Natives grabbed one too. He was tall and skinny with long black hair. I began to shoot baskets, and on my left were all four white boys, lined up against the wall. One of the whites was tall and large. All of the other whites were average in height. I was underneath the basketball hoop, and that's when it happened. One of the Natives threw a basketball at me, hitting my head. I moved out of the way, and he swung on me, hitting me right in my mouth. I could taste my blood, and it didn't taste good. My teeth felt like they caved in. My mouth was in serious pain. Then all four whites began to attack the Natives, and there was a large fight in the gym.

"Come on, bitch!"

"Let's go motherfucker!" They were talking to one another as they fought.

Both Natives were on the ground getting smashed

while I sat back watching it happen.

"Stay on the ground punk," the big white guy said.

Then out of nowhere six guards came flooding the gym, and there was blood all over the gym floor. It took all six guards to stop the fight that turned into a beating. I wish I would've known both groups were at war, but I didn't. How was I supposed to know something was going down? My teeth were in pain, and the fight was caught on camera. There was a camera at the top, right-hand corner of the ceiling. All four whites were placed in handcuffs, and both Natives were taken to the medical room. I was escorted to the medical room as well, but I was taken after the Natives. I was placed into a holding cell, and I waited until it was clear. I was eventually seen by the nurse. She was black and had black hair and brown eyes.

"You got hit in your mouth?"

"Yes," I said.

"Well you better leave your teeth alone," she said.

"They feel pretty loose," I said.

"There is really nothing I can do," she replied.

She was looking me over closely, and she was wearing blue medical gloves.

"Is he good to go back to his cell?"

The guard was present in the room, and he was

leaning against the wall.

"Ya, they reviewed the camera," he said. "And he didn't hit anyone."

The guard was tall and had blond hair with blue eyes. His name tag read *Patts*. I was escorted back to my unit, and my belongings were still outside of my cell door. The guard from the control tower popped my cell door, and I was let into my cell.

"Close the door behind you, Bower," Patts said.

I went into my cell and shut the door behind me. I went to lay down, and I noticed that I didn't have a cellmate. I was happy about it too. My teeth were in pain, and I tried not to close my mouth during my sleep. I laid on my mattress, and I wished the pain would go away. I was given no pain medication for my injury, and I laid on my mattress until I fell asleep.

Chapter 3 Confused

Dorothea Dix is the historic figure that changed the way people with mental illness were treated in America. Dix changed the way the system was ran. Which the old way was by placing those with mental illness into prisons, and jails instead of hospitals.

"Do you know the charges you're facing?"

Behind the glass was a folder with two large books that my attorney brought in. I was seated on the other side of the glass. I had a phone in my hand, while my attorney Mac had a phone in his hand.

"Austin, you are looking at a lot of time right now," Mac said. "A class two felony, which carries up to a two to fifty."

I looked across the glass staring at Mac.

"Can I have that time reduced?"

"You can accept a deal once I get one figured out for you," Mac said. "If I were you, I would take the deal if I can get one arranged. It would be in your best interest for your situation if you did."

I looked across at him staring again, because there was nowhere else to look.

"I won't make it in prison, Mac," I said.

"Well, this is your best chance at survival," Mac said as he began looking at his papers in his folder and shuffling them around.

"Well, let me see," Mac said. "Ya, Austin, it's your best shot, so I don't know what else to tell you. They already have a confession from you. Anything you plea now most likely won't help you."

Mac had on a blue tie and a gray suit. His hair was white from his old age. He had on silver glasses, and he kept his face clean. He was a little chubby as well —not fat, just chubby.

"I will ask the prosecutor to reduce the sentence," Mac said. "If I do and she agrees, would you take the deal?"

"Yes."

"Okay, then I will see what I can do for you."

"What about the other guy?"

"What other guy?"

"Hawkboy," I said.

"Austin," Mac said, "there is no one else in custody for this crime but you. I got your letters about it. You are the only one who is being charged right now. What did you tell the police about this other person?"

"I told them he robbed the guy," I said. "I also told them I didn't rob anyone. I did tell them that I was there though," I said.

36

"Okay, Austin," Mac said. "Well for right now I will work on a deal."

"That's it?"

"For now," Mac said.

As Mac began to pack up his books and belongings, I waited for the guard to let me out. As I waited for the guard to let me out, I watched them through the window in the control tower.

"Okay, Bower, are you all set?"

The voice projected out of the small, silver, square box with little dots on it.

"Yes, I am good to go," I said.

"Fantastic," the guard said with a hint of sarcasm.

The door popped and I was headed back to my cell to wait for lunch. The meals were often cold and wet, or cold and dry. I hated the food nonetheless. I had a cell that was small and also empty, littered with trash. I had paper all over the ground. And the light remained on all throughout the night. Sleep was uneasy for the most part, restless. I often tossed and turned throughout the night. I had fears that would come in my mind all of the time. I had to get away, I thought. I needed to escape this madness. My cell number read A-nineteen on the outside of my cell. I had no cellmate at the time. My mind would race more than I enjoyed. So having no cellmate made things easier for me. The unit I was on was general population. I came out with about twenty to twenty-nine other inmates. It varied from time to time. There were no televisions on the unit that I was on. My unit was admissions. It was the first step before an inmate would be classified, which the other classifications were B, C, and D units. D was maximum security, and C and B were minimum and medium security. I was on A unit, which you have a mixture of inmates ranging from murder to theft. I saw inmates come and go quite often. I kept thinking to myself, *I wish that could be me leaving right now.* I had no radio or money to buy a radio for that matter. As I sat on my bed, I often wondered who I would fight, if I would fight at all. If a fight would even happen. Things that were uncertain to me. As I thought this thought, my door began to pop open as did all the other doors. The guards didn't radio when it was time for rec. They just popped all the doors, leaving it up to the inmate to figure it out. Chatter began to break out like the plague. I saw inmates walking up to one another to talk. Some would pull out their decks of playing cards. Others would trade store items for envelopes. Many things would happen. Some would go up to shower with their towels and wash cloths along with their shampoo and soap. I had a few people come up to me, and it made me feel uncomfortable. However at this time I was in better shape. I was healthy. I was young and agile. I was only twenty years old. Fresh, new, brand new. I was cut and lean with a six pack untouched. I had a good build for my frame. My defense was the fact I looked like I could fight. If I could, that was a different story. I knew that I couldn't, and I knew it all too well.

"So what charges are you facing?"

He was short and had a medium build with brown hair and brown eyes. He was white, and he was standing by a white pillar near the control tower.

"Robbery," I said.

"Who did you rob?"

"No one," I said.

"Ya, we're all innocent," he said.

He looked away briefly.

"My name is Kregg by the way. I'm here on some petty bullshit."

"Ya, like what?"

"I had weed on me when I got pulled over by the police. My dumb ass let them search my vehicle, and wallah here I am," he said.

"That sucks."

"Well not as much as your situation. I'm not here for robbing no one, like you. I feel for you, kid."

"Thanks," I said.

"So you took a hit?" He was referring to the fight

earlier.

"Ya."

"How do your teeth feel?"

"They hurt."

"I bet they do," he said. "You'll be good though."

"How do you mean?"

"Your mouth will heal up," he said.

He moved on to another subject.

"So do you want to play some cards?"

"Sure."

I followed Kregg to a nearby table where two of his friends were already seated.

"Hey guys, this is...." Kregg paused, waiting for me to talk.

"Austin," I said.

"Austin," Kregg said. "He wants to play some cards with the gang."

"Well, Austin, come take a seat. We play spades at this table."

The two other men were white with blond hair. Both of them looked like brothers. Same facial description, same everything. It's just one of them had bigger arms than the other.

"Are you both brothers?"

"No," the one on the right said. "Why, do we look like brothers?"

"Yes," I said.

"Ya, we're brothers," the one on the right said with a smile.

"Hey, I'm John, and this is my brother Tim," John said.

They were both laughing while they spoke.

"Are you pulling my leg now?"

"No seriously, we are brothers," Tim said.

"Oh, okay." I had a hard time believing the both of them.

I sat down, and we began to play spades. Tim was the one who dealt the cards.

We played teams, and I was on Kregg's team. Both brothers played on the same team. We played all the way until lunch was called, and we had to lock down before we ate. It was some dumb rule we had to follow. As I was in my room, I waited for the central control officer to pop my door. He did eventually. Everyone came rushing out trying to be first in line and trying to survive. Other inmates trying to hustle slower inmates. As a matter of fact, some tried to hustle me. Tim from the card game earlier came up to me to do just that.

.

"Hey Austin, I bet you if we win the game after chow, then I get your lunch for tomorrow," Tim said.

He had a cocky attitude to him.

"Deal," I said. "And if we win, I get your lunch tomorrow."

He looked at me briefly.

"All right, you got yourself a deal there," he said.

I sat down to wait until the line died down for me to grab my tray. The line seemed longer than what it should be. The officers did the passing out of the trays. There were two officers passing out the meals, both female officers. Both were attractive too. One tall with long blond hair and a nice build. The other was short with a nice build. The shorter one had brownish blond hair, and she had a cute face. The meal looked nasty; it looked like something made up from garbage. It was disgusting for sure. And I saw flies hovering over the meals. They looked to be fruit flies of some sort. Almost like gnats. I went up to the chow line to get my food, and I grabbed my tray. The food looked mushy and distasteful. I had no choice but to eat it though if I wanted to survive. I went to sit down with Tim, John and Kregg. The four of us had a thing going on, almost like we would look out for one another if something were to go down. All four of us were white. They knew the drill. I didn't necessarily really know. I had never really been in an all out fist fight before other than in high school, and that was hardly a fight at all. I didn't think I would survive prison simply because I have autism. That factor alone would make it a challenge. So I ate my food and then dumped my tray. From there we were all instructed to go back to our cells.

I was still alone, and I was afraid of going to prison. I had a lot on my mind. That is without question. So it had gotten late, and lunch and dinner had passed. I decided to take my bedding and end my life before prison ended me. I took all my white sheets, and I tied them under my desk. Then I tied them around my throat, and I laid flat on the ground with my head facing the floor. The gravity caused me to have all my weight from my legs go back against my neck. I laid there for nearly two minutes, and then I saw small specks of blood coming out of my nose from the pressure. I started to panic. I tried to yell for help, but I couldn't; my throat wouldn't let me. What happened was spit came drooling out of my mouth. I heard the door to the unit open and close, and all of a sudden a guard doing rounds saw me attempting to commit suicide.

"Oh shit! Run nineteen!" He became frantic in a hurry.

"God dammit run nineteen right now!"

He was yelling on his radio.

"It's an emergency!"

He continued to yell.

The guard was trying to save my life. But I wanted to die, and I'd rather die than go to prison. The guard began to shake the door trying to get it open.

"Run nineteen!" This time the guard sounded scared.

He finally got the door to open, and afterwards he ran in. He took a knee next to my head placing his hands on me. He began to unravel the sheets. He had to do it one by one, because of how I had fashioned them. A team of guards came in one after another with a nurse. The nurse did an evaluation on me. The nurse saw the blood dripping down my nose. The guard finally had me in an upright position. I was siting on the floor with my legs pointing out. I began to cry and weep. Tears were flowing down my face.

 After I recovered, the guards had me moved to booking.

The guards carried me with their hands, dragging my feet on the floor as they carried me away. These guards were pretty strong.

"Damn Bower, you really wanted to die?"

There were too many guards around to make out which one was which.

I was carried all the way to booking, and I was placed in a cell that had a chair with straps on it. The chair looked like it tilted back a little. The chair was made out of hard plastic. I was forced in the chair and tied down to the straps. Legs, arms, and chest. I was seated in the chair for over thirty minutes yelling and screaming to let me out of the chair. I was angry that I was forced to be in this chair. I began to cry.

The room smelt like urine and poop. The walls had gang markings all over them.

The floor was a greenish gray color that looked like vomit, and the chair was so uncomfortable. I was afraid for my life, and I was afraid for my future. I was acting like a coward.

My future?

What future? I thought to myself.

There was a glass window with guards standing on the other side of it. The window appeared to be a plastic glass. Strong and unbreakable to punches.

The floor to the cell that I was in had a hole that inmates would pee and poop in.

I was going mad being strapped to this chair, and it felt as if my back were bending.

I was in pain for sure, and these fuckers knew it too. They fucking knew it all along while they watched me laughing. They stared at me laughing.

"Look at Bower in pain!"

"Bower, is it tight enough for you?"

There were about six to seven guards outside by the window of my cell.

Joking and laughing at my pain.

"Let me out of here, dammit. Let me out of here right fucking now, you motherfuckers! You mother fucking sons of bitches, let me out of here right now!"

Tears were falling down my face, and I was in physical pain.

I knew that I was all alone. I questioned God—why would he want this for me?

"Why would you want this for me God? I didn't rob that man," I pleaded. "I didn't do it."

All the while the guards were making jokes about me and how I was strapped in this God-forsaken chair. Then it got worse, and my anger intensified when I saw him. I grew silent when I saw him. It was the one and only Hawkboy. He was in cuffs a month after the crime, and I knew why he was here.

"Do you know if Austin Bower is here?"

The female guard pointed behind him toward me from the desk.

Why is he asking for my name?

He turned around, and he looked at me.

"Snitch, you fucking snitch!"

I remained quiet, and I said nothing at all.

Why would he ask for my name from the guards? I

thought.

As Hawkboy began yelling, they escorted Hawkboy out of booking.

A lady in a black suit came in to speak with me. She had a key to open the cell block.

The door made an odd noise when she opened it. It was like rusted metal grinding.

"Okay, Mr. Bower, let's start with a talk ," Sherry said. "My name is counselor Sherry Cord. You probably didn't know this, but I used to work with your father. I am sorry about his passing, and I know that was probably hard on you. He was a good man."

"Ya," I said.

"Ya," she said.

She was eye level with me, and there was a moment of silence.

"Well, Austin, we will be sending you to the crisis center, where they will undergo an evaluation on you," she said. "Make sure you cooperate to the best of your abilities, and we will help you as much as we can."

"Okay," I replied.

Sherry exited and closed the door behind her.

I remained on the very uncomfortable chair for the next half an hour.

Then, after the wait of excruciating pain, a guard with a gold badge and a guard with a silver badge came into the cell. They both placed me in full body restraints.

I was placed in a belly chain, ankle cuffs, and handcuffs. After they had chained me up, I was escorted through two large metal doors, which led to an elevator. From the elevator the scene changed into a lower level parking lot. The parking lot was downtown, and it had high security. I was led to a van, which was a county vehicle. I was led to the backseat and the ramp. It was dark in the parking garage, only a few lights were on. I was asked to get into the backseat and to watch my step.

"Okay, Bower, let's roll," the guard said after buckling my seat belt for me.

I figured the one with the gold badge was the sergeant or the lieutenant.

The other guard was obviously a lower rank than he was.

Both guards climbed into the van, and off we were. We exited out of the parking garage and onto the busy street. The ride was quiet and smooth, and it was dark outside and the stars were shining.

It was mid-September, and the sky had only a few clouds.

My mind began to wander, and I was facing a lot of

time.

Fifty years is a long long time, I thought.

If I received the entire fifty, I wouldn't be out until I was in my seventies.

We traveled and the ride seemed to be unending.

I thought to myself how nice it would be just to keep driving.

I'd rather drive around until my sentence is up.

Then we arrived to my next destination, which was the Lincoln Crisis Center.

I was escorted by the two guards out of the van.

"Okay, Bower, we're here," the guard in front said.

One walked behind me, and the other walked in front of me. The guard with the gold badge had brown hair. He was very skinny and tall, not like the other one. The other guard had a large belly.

The sergeant was speaking through the microphone on the door.

I assumed he was the sergeant. The door popped, and I was led in by the two guards, who walked me to an elevator. They both made sure the door was locked behind us before we advanced forward.

Once we arrived at the elevator, the elevator opened. The elevator smelled weird like chemicals or something like bleach. We then came out of the

49

elevator in front of another large door. While we were on the second floor, we waited outside. The guard began removing my belly chain and cuffs. There was no small talk or conversation. I remained standing still until I was greeted by a black woman and escorted inside.

Chapter 4 *In Crisis*

Dorothea Dix was born April 4, 1802. She led the nation with the movement for better care for the mentally ill, and she died July 18, 1887.

The crisis center had many rooms to its one unit. It was in fact only one unit, if I may add. There was a television room and a small dining room. There was a shower room that techs had access to with a key. The rooms were all single bedded rooms. The unit was co-ed. Women were mixed with men on the unit. However, the staff and doctors tolerated no mistrust between the men and women. No women were to go into the men's rooms, and no men were to go into the women's rooms. They were to stay separate from each other. And the way they did this best was by conducting ten minute checks. That is how the system was designed to keep order and safety.

I arrived at the crisis center late in the evening. It was about eight or nine o'clock at night once I had arrived. I was spoken to by a large black lady. She had curly hair and was very pretty. She was large, and even with that she was still pretty. I kept thinking I would stay at the crisis center until my sentence was all the way up. I still hadn't been sentenced yet, and the not knowing scared me deeply. I was terrified of what the judge would sentence me to.

"Austin, follow me," she said.

She led me into a back room that had one large desk and a vital kit. The kit included a thermometer and a blood pressure cuff. It also included a heart rate monitor.

"So, we need to do your intake," she said.

"Okay," I said.

"My name is Shawntell. I already know who you are," she said. "So, are you feeling suicidal?"

"Yes," I replied.

"Okay," she said. "Are you feeling like hurting anyone else?"

"No," I said.

"Very good. Who is your emergency contact?"

"My mom."

"Do you know her phone number?"

"Yes."

"What is it?"

"It's four zero two, five zero four, two nine nine one," I said.

"Okay, great. Do you have any brothers or sisters?"

"Yes," I said.

"Okay, how many?"

"I have four siblings all together," I said. "I have an older brother, and two younger brothers, and a baby sister."

"Okay, great."

I was feeling hungry, and I wanted some food. My stomach was growling; however, I was a little hesitant to even ask for food.

"Hey Shawntell," I said, "Can I please have some food? I am pretty hungry." I figured she would say no.

"Ya, sure we can get you something. I just need to take your vitals first," she said.

Wow, she caught me by surprise, I thought.

"Let's get this cuff around your arm here," she said. "Wow, do you work out? You have pretty big arms."

"Ya, I do a lot of push ups," I said.

"I can tell."

As she began trying to fit one of the cuffs around my arm, she was having a difficult time doing so.

"You know what? I will need to use the bigger cuff on you, 'cause this one isn't going to work," she said.

She began looking for a bigger cuff to place on my arm. As she was looking, I was focused on the room.

53

The walls were white, and the carpet was blue. I noticed there were some inspirational pictures hanging up too.

"Follow your dreams" it read, and it had a picture of an Olympic swimmer on it. The swimmers head was coming up for air out of the water gasping. The swimmer had goggles on, along with a swimming cap.

"Okay, I have a bigger cuff."

"Okay," I said.

"So, Austin, where are you originally from?"

She was standing now.

"I'm from California," I said.

"Born?"

"Yes."

"Did you enjoy it at all?"

"Yes. However, it was dangerous," I said.

"How so?" She stood over me in question.

"Shootings and riots," I said.

"Really?" Her eyelids rose, and I noticed she seemed surprised by this.

"Ya, it got worse after the police assaulted King and walked," I said.

"Walked?"

"Beat the charges," I said.

"Oh, walked, gotcha," she said. "I didn't understand what you meant at first."

As she was putting the cuff away, she was in the process of grabbing the thermometer as well. She was in front of me, and I could see the cleavage of her chest. She also had a low-cut shirt on. Since the color of her shirt was blue, it mixed well with her complexion.

"Here we go, Austin," she said. "We have cheese crackers, and we have some yogurt.

"Okay, can I have both?"

"Sure, why not," she said.

I began to eat my snacks. I was hungry, and I didn't take my time either. As I ate, Shawntell sat across from me, finishing up her paperwork. She would occasionally look up to smile at me. She was pretty, and it didn't bother me that she was black. Her size didn't make her ugly either. As I finished my snacks one by one, Shawntell looked at me and stood up.

"Austin, let me show you where your room is," she said.

She instructed me to follow her and I began to walk behind her in a line. She led me down a long hallway. I saw two other patients standing by their doors. One male and one female. I saw no other staff nearby. At least I thought no other staff was nearby. Shawntell led me by a cage that was surrounded by glass. The cage had a solid door to it that needed a key to get in and out of. Shawntell led me to a room near a small library room. The small library room had two chairs and four bookshelves all included in the library. For it being so small, it had a lot of books I thought.

"This is our library," Shawntell said. "You can select a book anytime you would like. You can also relax in one of these comfortable chairs whenever you would like," she said.

I walked into the room and I saw tons of books. Some appeared to never have been touched. I noticed a few mystery books and a few history books as well.

"Your room will be right next to the library," she said. "Here, come with me."

I began to follower her, and I noticed a large hallway wall with a large painting on the wall. The painting read many different things like "Honor and respect." There were many colors on the wall.

Shawntell led me to a television room.

"This is the television room," she said. "You can pick out a movie to watch if you want or you can simply watch a television show if you want to."

I saw three patients sitting in wood padded chairs, and they were all fixated on the television. Their heads turned slightly to look at me when I came in. I noticed about twelve chairs that were in the television room. The television room had one glass window to it. Shawntell caught my attention, and she asked me to follow her into the next room.

"This is the dining room where we have breakfast, lunch, and diner," she said. "We also have late night snacks in this room too."

"Okay," I said.

"Here, let me show you where you can make a phone call," she said.

She led me back the way we had originally came from. Past the library and past the cage. As I was walking past the cage, I saw lots of paperwork in files and in cabinets. I also saw two computers and a room that led even further back than the cage itself. Shawntell led me to two desks that had phone jacks installed in them.

"Okay, this is how this works, Austin," she said. "You can ask us for the phone, and we will provide it as long as it is during normal phone hours. You can dial your own number, but we can disconnect your line if the person you call doesn't want to talk to you.

"Okay," I responded respectfully.

"Okay, perfect," she said. "Now since that is out of the way, I can go get you your bedding. By the way, phone times are tomorrow. It's too late to make a call now, if you were wondering."

"Okay," I said.

I then saw two other staff come on to the unit. One was a tall blond haired women. The other was a short, skinny women. Both of them looked like they exercised.

"Hi, you must be Austin. My name is Bonka," she said.

She had an accent to her voice. She sounded German, or possibly Russian. I couldn't quite figure her accent out, and she also wore glasses. The other tech introduced herself as Maggen. She was shorter than Bonka, and she moved in grace as she walked.

"So when will I see the doctor?"

"Probably tomorrow," Bonka said. "It's after hours right now, so no one is here."

"Okay."

"Here, let's get you your medications, Austin," Maggen said. "The nurse should be back any minute."

"You can wait over here to get your meds," Bonka said.

"Okay."

I took a seat near the desks where the phone jacks were. The desk was near the nurses' station. I waited for the nurse to show. I sat in the chair that was made of plastic for the next ten minutes. The staff eventually left, and the nurse eventually showed up.

"Hi, you must be Austin. I am Nurse Len," she said.

She was larger than I was. She wore glasses and had curly brown hair. She wore a white lab coat with bunnies on it.

"Let me get set up here," she said.

She began to open the wooden door, and she closed it behind her. The door had a double contraption to it. The bottom remained locked when the top was open.

"Okay, let's get started," she said.

"Okay."

"Now the doctor ordered you three different medications," she said. "Those meds are Geodon, Abilify, and Depakote.

"Are you sure? Because I am allergic to Depakote," I said.

"Ya, it says it right here," she said.

"Well, I'm not going to take it," I said. "That medication caused me liver complications as a child.

"Okay," she said carelessly. "We will just mark you down as a refusal then."

"I'm not refusing anything," I said. "Change the order."

"I can't."

"Why not?"

"Because the order has to be done by a doctor," she said.

"What the heck!"

"I know it seems unfair, but we need you to take your pills, Austin."

"Even after I just told you I am allergic to the Depakote, you still want me to take it? What kind of shit is that?"

More staff began to approach me, and they were not backing off.

"Austin, we need you to calm down," Bonka said.

"I am calm, don't you dare tell me to calm down!"

I was becoming aggravated. I knew that if I didn't calm down nothing good would come out of it.

"Okay, I will take my medications," I said.

"Okay," the nurse said.

"Are we good now?" Bonka was asking.

"Yes, I am good," I said.

I took the medication that was in the cup, and I swallowed them with the water that the nurse gave to me. It had gotten late, and it was already ten o'clock at night. I had my meds, and I was starting to get tired. I was afraid of the Depakote messing up my liver again. I thought this was awful. I did not like this at all. I went to my room, and I noticed that my bed was already made up for me. I climbed into bed, and I began to drowse off into sleep. It was a long day. I just came from the county jail, and I didn't know what I was going to do. I still hadn't seen my judge yet. A month had passed, and I still hadn't seen my mother yet. I wanted things to get better. Things were bad right now, really bad. I just didn't know where my life was headed, I thought to myself. As I fell asleep, it seemed like sleep was my only escape from this living nightmare.

Chapter 5 *Still in Crisis*

America has returned to it's old ways of how the mentally ill are treated. In 2017 studies have shown America has now returned to the ways of the 1840's.

I had been in the crisis center for just a few days. The food was garbage, and the coffee they had was weak. The food was brought over through the county jail. I saw the cart that it was carried on. The cart had a hatch device on it, and the cart read 'Property of the Lincoln County Corrections.' I was in the dining room writing a letter to my attorney trying to figure things out. I knew that Hawkboy was now in lock up, and I didn't know if he was telling or not. I questioned it because of his behavior towards me. He didn't even know what I had said, and yet he was calling me a snitch. That brought me to believe that he was telling on me. I just had a gut feeling on it. I didn't trust him anyways even though I thought he was my friend. He claimed to be my friend and that we were going to a party. Yet he decided to rob someone. And he wanted to take me down with him. I knew very little about Hawkboy. I just assumed he was telling, but about what? He was the one who did it. I know he was caught for the shoe too. I knew because that is all he could complain about was his shoe falling off. He wouldn't stop complaining either; he was like a gnat in my ear. I was writing a letter to my attorney trying to get as much help as I could. After I wrote the letter, I decided to call my mother to let her know where I was at.

"Mom!"

"How are you doing?"

"Where are you, Mom?"

I was so happy to hear her voice.

"I'm okay," she said. "I am at work right now."

"Mom, it wasn't me who robbed that guy," I said.

"Austin!" I could tell she was upset. "I don't know what happened," she said.

"You believe me though, don't you?"

"I don't know what I believe right now," she said. "That's not my focus right now though. My focus is on helping you as much as possible."

"Okay."

"Do you have a mental health board hearing coming up soon?"

"What is that? I don't know what that is," I said.

"Never mind, I can call and ask them," she said.

"Can you visit me tonight?"

63

"What time?"

"Seven," I said.

"No, I will be with your brother," she said.

"Okay, what about this Thursday?" I was eager to have a visit.

"Thursday?"

"Ya, visiting days are Tuesday, Thursday, and Saturday."

"What time Saturday?"

"I'm not sure. I think there is one in the afternoon, and seven o'clock at night," I said.

"Okay, I can do the seven o'clock one this Saturday," she said.

"Okay great, I will see you this Saturday, Mom. I love you, Mom."

"I love you too, honey."

I hung up the phone and headed to the bathroom. The sinks were made of metal, and the mirrors were metal as well. The toilets were metal too, with metal buttons that flushed the toilet. There were two dividers between the toilet seats. There was a stall for pooping and a stall for urinating. I used the bathroom, and I walked over to the sink. I looked at myself in the mirror, and I began to cry. I cried my eyes out because I didn't want to be here anymore. All of a sudden a patient walked in while I was crying. The door swung open. I discontinued my sobbing, and I exited the bathroom. As I walked out I saw a man dressed in a nice outfit. His outfit looked to be a button shirt with a pair of slacks and a pair of dress shoes.

"Hi, are you Austin?"

"Yes, I am Austin," I said.

"Great, let me meet with you if you have a moment," he said. "I am Doctor Jerry. I am the psychologist here at the wonderful crisis center. I will need you to fill these forms out."

The doctor handed me a small pack of papers.

"These are all part of your evaluation," he said. "Take your time on them, and don't rush."

He wore a pair of black glasses, and he also had gray curly hair.

"You will meet with the crisis center psychiatrist later today," he said.

"What is his name?"

"His name is Doctor Corey," he said. "He will do a great job with treating you fair."

"Okay, thank you," I said.

Doctor Jerry handed me the papers, and I went to the desk where a pencil was already present. And I began to do my written evaluation. The evaluation asked me weird questions such as:

65

'Have you been depressed in the last month?'

There were other questions as well. Such as:

'Do you feel like hurting others?'

I figured this was mandatory to finish this assignment. I didn't want to, but I did it anyways. I kept thinking about my charges and how all this is going to impact my future. I didn't keep in account that I wasn't convicted yet. I should have, but I didn't. It's not like it made much of a difference anyways I thought. I was around a bunch of crazy people. I soon became discouraged as I filled in the blank circles. I was falling off track, and I noticed I began to gain weight from the Depikote. I felt like I may have gained five pounds, if not more, since I was on it. I was to meet with the doctor soon, and I had no idea if he was there to help or not. Doctor Jerry said he was, but I had no one else to ask.

I was uncertain on who was really here to help. I felt like I couldn't trust any of the staff. I started seeing things about their behavior and mannerisms that I didn't like. I noticed some of them would provoke other patients, and some of them wouldn't. It became apparent that not all of them could be trusted. I eventually finished the assignment, and it took me a little over an hour to finish. I went to the day room, and I handed in my assignment to the tech who was sitting down watching television. The movie *Apollo Thirteen* was being played, the film that had Tom

Hanks in it and Keven Bacon in it as well. It was a great film—too bad I had to watch it in the crisis center, I thought. Time went by, and I felt like I was in slow motion for the most part. When I didn't pay attention to the clock, time went by quickly. From watching movies on television to writing family and my attorney to eating the nasty food and drinking the watered down coffee, I just had enough of it, and I would lie down on my bed during the day doing absolutely nothing. One afternoon was extremely weird. I was writing my attorney, and an old lady came in the room. She had gray hair and wrinkled skin, and she looked to be in her seventies.

"I want a skinhead to fuck me," she said.

I was the only one in the dining room while I was writing my letter, and I did in fact have a shaved head, so I knew she was referring to me. I shaved my head with a Bic razor. I was going bald anyway, so it made things easier for me.

"I want a skinhead to fuck my old pussy right now," she said.

She began to take off her shirt and her pants. She was almost fully naked. She had white wrinkled skin. I saw her old breasts that looked like sandbags.

She began to yell even louder, "Fuck my pussy right now, you Nazi skinhead!"

I was blown away by this. I had never experienced anything like it before. I was scared and afraid of what she would do next. She climbed on the table completely naked, and she spread her legs open. I exited the room as soon as possible, and I told staff what was happening.

"This lady is naked! She is trying to have sex with me. I left as soon as possible," I said.

"Okay, we will handle it," they said.

Five techs went into the dining room to take care of the situation. The old women put up a fight too. She began to yell and scream.

"I want his dick! I want to be fucked!"

I went to my room to get as far away from her as I could. I kept thinking that the staff were going to accuse me of convincing her to take her clothing off, which I had not done at all. I was simply writing my letter to my attorney. I saw from my room that techs were taking the woman into the full bedroom, which is where a patient goes to be tied down if they are unsafe to themselves or others. I hadn't experienced that yet, and I hoped that I didn't have to experience it. I saw the room before, and it has straps that tie your arms and legs down, and even your chest. I for the most part stayed to myself, and I avoided others. I wanted this process to be done with and fast.

"Austin?"

"Yes?"

"I am Doctor Corey," he said.

"I thought you were going to meet with me on Tuesday," I said.

"That was the plan," he said. "I was called out to an emergency So here I am, and it's Friday."

"Better late than never," I said.

"Yes...yes...I suppose," he said. "Lets get started, shall we?

Doctor Corey was short and had gray hair. He wore glasses and had a hint of Switzerland in his voice. His tie did not meet the coordination of his suit. The brown made the black look very uneven, and his white shirt didn't help things either.

"You will have a mental health board hearing this coming Wednesday," he said.

"Okay."

"Can I bring you back to my office to ask you a few questions?"

"Sure," I said.

 "Follow me this way."

Doctor Corey nodded at a tech standing nearby. The tech was a male in a black dress shirt, and he wore slacks with brown shoes. His name was Calvin. Calvin, Doctor Corey, and I walked to his office, which we had to go through two locked doors to get to. He led me into his office, and it was dark with very little light from the sun that was peering through the window.

"Come take a seat," he said.

I sat down on a chair that was far more comfortable than the chairs in the television room of the crisis center.

"Do you know who you are?"

"Yes," I said.

"Do you know what the date today is?"

"I'm not sure," I said.

"Give me a guess," he said.

"October eighth, two thousand and nine," I said.

"Okay."

"What's your birth date?"

"August ninth, nineteen eighty-eight," I said.

"Okay."

He was writing down information on his paper.

"That is all we need here," he said.

He sounded like he had joy in his voice. Like he was ready to go to a Christmas party or something. Afterwards I was led back to the unit by Calvin, and I went through the motions all over again. The same routine—television, meals that sucked, and sleep. It was quite boring, and it taught me how to be lazy. I did this routine all the way until Saturday, the day I was able see my mother.

Chapter 6 The Visit

Nebraska is one of the only states that mix Civilly Committed Patients with Criminally Committed Patients in the United States.

Saturday was finally here. I was happy because I knew that I had a visit coming later in the evening. I woke up out of bed, and the techs cued me for breakfast. I was hungry, but I wasn't hungry for what they were serving. County jail food is no good. Take my word for it, and let that be a good enough reason not to have it. I walked from my room into the dining area. There were about fourteen patients in the dining room. I was number fifteen. I had come in last place, and all the good seats were taken. I was stuck next to this black-haired lady. She looked to be in her thirties. I sat next to her to eat. The staff brought me my tray, and the tray was different than the county jail trays. The meal consisted of cold hash browns and cold scrambled eggs. It was a small meal, and I would rather of had cereal than this garbage, I thought.

"Hi, I'm Molly. I like knives; do you like knives?"

I could tell she wasn't all there mentally.

"I also like big long dick's," she said.

She was very jittery.

"Do you have a big, long dick?"

"Molly!" The tech working the dining room snared.

"You need to stop doing that," John said.

The tech had a plaid shirt on. It was red with black stripes. He also had a pair of blue jeans on. His jeans were Levi's, I could tell. I wore Levi's in the community, that's how I knew. His shoes looked more like boots, and his hair was red. His face was thin and pale.

"I'm sorry," Molly said.

"So do you like pussy, or are you gay?"

"I'm not gay," I said.

"I don't know, you look pretty good to be straight," she said.

"Too good," she whispered.

"I would fuck you in a heartbeat," she said. "But I think your gay. I mean look at you; you look like a model."

"I am not gay!" I was very bothered by her comments.

"Okay, that's it, Molly. We need to move you," John said.

The techs helped escort Molly to another table, and as they were moving Molly, she winked at me. Her

73

back was turned to me. The techs moved Molly and exchanged her for another patient. I was sitting with an older man now. He looked to be in his fifties.

"So why are you here?"

I was just finishing my hash browns.

"I am here on something I didn't do," I said.

"You didn't do what?" He began questioning me closely.

"I didn't do the crime," I said.

"What was the crime?"

"Robbery."

"Oh, who did you rob?"

"No one," I said. "I told you I didn't do it."

"Ya...ya, we're all innocent," he said.

"No seriously, I didn't do it."

"Then who did do it?"

"I don't know," I said, "but it wasn't me!"

"Austin, you need to calm down," John said.

"Tell this old person to leave me alone then."

"What did he say to you?"

"Just tell him to leave me alone please," I said.

"Just tell me what he said."

"No, I'm not going to tell you what he said!"

"Okay, do you need to go to the quiet room?"

"No, I will calm down," I said.

"Okay, then just finish your breakfast, and later watch some television," he said.

"Okay."

I finished my tray and my milk, and I was headed to the television room. I laid low the rest of the day because of all the unwanted attention I had now. I knew all this visibility wasn't good for me, so I decided to stick to myself, which was harder than I initially thought. I thought it would be easy, but it wasn't. All through my stay women were coming to me with all types of lines. I just wasn't feeling it—I mean I was in the crisis center. This was not the place to hook up, and even I knew that. I wanted space from all of these people. I didn't want to be around all of these crazies. I felt like I couldn't get away, and I felt like I was trapped. I just wanted to see my mom, that is all I wanted. I wanted nothing more than to receive a hug from my mother. Time went bye, and I had lunch and dinner. It was past six o'clock now. I counted down every last minute and every last hour. I went to the bathroom to brush my teeth and put on deodorant. After I did my hygiene, I went to my room to wait. The tech working was Bonka, the one with the German accent, or possibly Russian. I wasn't sure where she was from, I just knew that I liked her.

"Austin, your mom is here to see you," Bonka said.

I was so happy. I couldn't wait to tell her how awful things were. I had a nice shirt on, not a dress shirt, but it was nice. I followed Bonka through two doors and down a long hallway. I entered into the room.

"Mom!"

"Hey, honey!"

She had on blue jeans and a button up shirt. My mom had curly hair, and her eyes were green. She wore white K-Swiss tennis shoes.

"How are you doing?"

"Not so good; it is awful here, and the food is garbage, and the shower has cold pressure."

"I am sorry to hear that," she said.

I could hear the sincerity in her voice. The room had a section of toys in the corner, and a camera was at the top right corner of the room. There were about ten chairs in the room, and a large window against the back wall.

"Here, I brought you some candies," she said.

"Thanks, Mom."

The candies were gushy and sweet, and as I ate we talked about how her home life was. I talked to my mom about her car and house. I also told my mom my fears.

"I think I'm going to go to prison, Mom," I said.

"Austin, I want you to know, I will not let you go to prison," she said. "Stop worrying."

"I can't Mom. Don't you see I'm afraid?"

"Yes, I see that you are afraid, but you must give it over to God," she said.

"Mom, they have me on depikote," I said.

"Who has you on depikote?"

She was surprised by my words.

"Doctor Corey," I said.

"Okay, I will see what I can do about that. You shouldn't be on that. It made your liver grow when you were younger," she said.

"That is what I told the nurse," I said. "But she wasn't listening."

"Ya, I will see what I can do," she said.

Bonka sat across from my mom and me reading a magazine. She was only there because she had to be. Time seemed to slip through our fingertips as our visit neared its end.

"Okay," Bonka said. "It's that time."

"Okay, I love you, Mom."

"I love you too, Austin."

"I will see you later, Mom."

I gave my mother a hug, and I wished her a good night. I was left in the room with Bonka. We waited until my mother was gone through the visiting doors. Bonka escorted me back, and I was happy, but only for a moment. I was stuck here with all these people that I didn't like. I took my medications, and I noticed I was gaining more weight too. I gained about fifteen pounds. I was sure it was from the poor food diet, and the medication and lack of exercise. There was an exercise room though, and it had a stationary bike and some pull down weights. It had no free weights at all, which was probably for safety reasons. I walked past the exercise room and back to the unit. I took my medication, and I was off to bed.

Chapter 7 Mental Health Board

The mental health crisis in America can be resolved if the political will is there to make the change.

I was still in the crisis center, and I was hoping I would wake up to my mom's house. However, I woke up to being around these crazy people and the hospital techs who worked with them. Young men my age were supposed to be going to school or playing sports. Young men my age were supposed to have a sane girlfriend to make love with, and I had neither of the three. Well counting a job, so four things I should have been doing. I wanted to work, and I wanted to get paid for my honest day's wage. Yet I was trapped in this horrifying facility, and I hated it. After waking I went to have breakfast, and it was the same old nasty breakfast from the days before. The same exact thing—it seemed to always be the same kind of breakfast. Cold or wet, and either way it wasn't any good. It wasn't the same as Mom's cooking, that's for sure. I went through the same routine as I had for the past two weeks. Today, though, I had a mental health board hearing.

Today was Wednesday, and October was approaching. I grabbed my clothing and a towel and a wash cloth, and I headed to the shower. I had shampoo and soap in my hand given to me by the tech. The tech who gave it to me was a bald black man, and his name was Kelly, and he told me that he was from New York. We spoke in conversation a few times, and we talked in the library and the dining room. He seemed to be a nice man who cared. I knew one thing about him, he always smiled at me, and that made me feel like a good person. Like I was accepted or respected, and I felt loved by him. His smile was caring, and I could tell that it was sincere. Kelly led me to the shower, and he unlocked the shower door for me. The shower door swung shut on its own, so you needed to hold it open after you unlocked it. It was like a fire safety door. The door was large, and it was made of wood. Near the door were long windows in the hallway. The shower door was located in the hallway near the front of the entrance of the crisis center. There were two shower rooms, and they both had separate doors. One was on the left, and the other one was on the right.

The one on the right was the good shower with hot water, and the one on the left was the bad shower with cold water. Someone was already in the good shower. It was this girl named Misty who had cut her forearm all the way open so that she would need stitches to help the wound. It was more like staples. I know because I saw them, and the cut was deep. Very deep in fact, and I don't know if she was in real pain emotionally or spiritually for that matter.

All that I did know was that this wound looked bad, and I mean horrific. I thought I had seen it all before, but this was real. I was able to see some of her scar tissue and even her muscle. That is how deep this wound was. I thought it looked like something out of a knife fight. The only difference was that she did it to herself, and someone else didn't do it to her. I only know this because she told me.

"I was raped," she said. "I feel so numb."

"Everything was stolen from me in those five minutes," she said. "Now I just think about dying."

I saw her pain, and her pain looked real in her eyes. It is scary to think another person's actions can lead you to such pain.

"Here you go, Austin," Kelly said. "Enjoy your shower."

Kelly said this with a smile on his face, not provoking and not instigating. His smile was genuine. The shower room was small, and there was no place to lay my clothing down. I had no choice but to place my laundry on the ground. I was bothered by this every time I used the shower at the crisis center. It made me feel inhuman, to know I was so low that I couldn't even have a place to hang my laundry. So as I turned the water on the pressure was automatic. The water rushed out hard, and it seemed to be dry rather than damp. I was hit so hard by the water that it didn't even give time to stay on my skin.

It was as if it hit me and then just bounced off. My skin would turn red, and sometimes I would even form bruises from the water pressure.

My clothes were all the way in the corner of the shower room. The water from the shower wouldn't even enter the drain if I may add. It was as if it went over the drain and then on to my clothes. My shower took nearly ten minutes, and the water was cold the entire time. I finished up, and I grabbed my clothing from the ground. My boxers were damp by the cold water. *Great*, I thought, *now I have wet boxers to wear. It would be nice to even have a chair.* I must be that low of a being to these people, and I couldn't shake it out of my head. I was lower than scum to this administration. With the exception of Kelly and a few others, I was lower than scum to the rest. I finished my shower, and I dried off my bruised arms. I then went back to my room, and it was still early yet, and nothing to really do. I was wide awake, and I wanted to play basketball. I wanted nothing else but to shoot hoops. I couldn't even do that. I laid in bed for another two hours until lunch was called. I walked past the old lady who wanted to have sex with me desperately. I entered the room, and I saw Misty and a few others waiting for their lunch. The room was bright, and it had round tables in it. The tables had four chairs a piece. There was a counter in the dining room, which had a sink connected to it. In the way back of the chow room there was also a camera in a square box. It was designed that way so no one could break the box and destroy the camera. I sat down at Misty's table, and there were two other guys sitting with her. Misty had a tattoo of stars on her face, and she was rather pretty. After she had told me her story I had no lustful thoughts for her. Instead I felt sorrow for her and her situation.

"Hey, Austin," she said.

She had a smile on.

"Hi."

"When are you getting out of here?"

"I don't know. Soon I hope."

"Ya, I'm pretty sure we all want to get out of here soon," she said.

The room was dry. I felt like I could have a nose bleed at any second.

"Ya, this place sucks," I said.

"You're telling me."

The younger man at the table began to speak.

He was new to the crisis center. I could tell, because I hadn't seen him before.

"What's your name?"

The young man had on a blue shirt that said *'Rock your heart out'*. He had glasses and a haircut that was shaggy. He was white, and thin, and his teeth were yellow.

"Chris," he said.

"Hi, I am Austin," I said.

"I gathered that."

He had some sass to himself.

"So why are you here?"

"I am here for having sex with someone," he said.

"Really? They locked you up for that?"

"Ya, I guess," he said.

"Was it with a minor?"

"I rather not say," he said.

"No, do tell," I said.

"No, I rather not," he said.

Misty slowly moved away from him, and I followed Misty to the table across from Chris. Me and Misty were sitting by ourselves now. Misty and I were both quiet; and I didn't want to say anything to Misty. I felt like anything would set her off. So I sat there with my mouth shut, and I can tell something triggered her. I remained quiet until lunch arrived. I ate my food, and I drank the tea they gave us. Kelly was the one who served us our meal. I went to the television room after I was done eating, and a man with a black striped suit came in to see me.

"Austin?"

"Yes, I am Austin," I said.

"Hey, I am your mental health public defender," he said. "My name is Mr. Tate. Can I speak with you somewhere private?"

"Sure," I said.

I followed Mr. Tate to the back room of the unit, near the exercise station. I noticed that Mr. Tate had some nice dress shoes on.

"Do you need to be let in?" Kelly was asking Mr. Tate. "I got it, Kelly," Jim said. "Hi, I am Jim."

Jim was introducing himself to Mr. Tate, and Jim had curly black hair and a small nose. His voice was hoarse, and he sounded sick. That or he just had a yelling match with someone. Jim was wearing a white dress shirt and black slacks.

"Here you go," Jim said.

I followed Mr. Tate into the back room. There was a long table and many chairs that surrounded the table.

"Well today you have a hearing," he said.

I was sitting down while he was talking.

"I want to ask you a few questions, Austin. Do you feel unsafe to yourself and to others?"

"Yes," I said.

"Do you feel that you need to go to a higher level of care?"

85

"Yes?"

I said yes slowly, and I sounded uncertain.

"If you don't, tell me now," he said.

"No, I do feel I need a higher level of care."

I would say anything to survive, I thought.

"What's this meeting like?"

"Your mental health hearing?"

"Yes," I said.

"Well, there are three judges who will decide if you need a higher level of care," he said.

"Those Judges are attorneys or workers in the community," he said.

"Okay," I said.

"Your meeting is in about thirty minutes."

"Well, I need you to get a hold of my mother."

"Why?"

"Because my mom wants to be there," I said.

"Okay, what is your mom's name?"

"Brenda," I said.

"Okay."

Mr. Tate pulled out his pen and began writing on his yellow legal pad.

"Whats your mom's phone number?"

"Four zero two," I said, "five zero four, two nine nine one."

"Okay, I will try and get a hold of her," he said. "Is your mother your legal guardian?"

"What's that?"

"Someone appointed by the courts to take care of you and make decisions for you," he said.

"No, she is not my legal guardian."

"Okay, well I will call her anyways and see what I can do," he said.

"Okay, thank you."

As he began to stand up, we were both leaving the room.

"Okay, I will give your mom a call, and I will see you in thirty minutes or so. I will have you come back with me when the time comes," he said.

"Okay. Mr. Tate," I stopped him briefly before he walked away.

"Yes."

"I don't want to go to prison," I said.

"Okay. This is not prison we would be sending you to," he said. "It is a hospital."

"Okay," I said.

I walked back to the unit's television room. They had a movie on, and the room was dark because a patient wanted the lights off. I sat down and relaxed myself to watch a movie with a few other people in the room. Kelly and Jim were both seated watching the movie *Dead Poets Society*. Kelly had a clip board in his hand because he was on ten minute checks. When a staff member was on checks, every ten minutes they had to walk around the unit to keep track of all the patients and to also insure they were safe, and simply not dead. I sat down watching this movie thinking to myself how sad it wa that the main character kills himself in the end. I waited until Mr. Tate came back to get me. I watched as Kelly got up to do his checks, and Jim stayed seated watching the television. Jim was laughing, and I was just staring at him, thinking he was laughing for no good reason. I watched as Mr. Tate came back to the unit, and I saw him through the glass window.

"Okay Austin, we are ready for you," Mr. Tate said.

I began to walk with Mr. Tate.

"Your mom is here, just so you know."

I smiled at that news, and Mr. Tate led me through three different doors. His badge allowed him to have access to go through them all without a key. I walked into the room, and Mr. Tate led me to a chair.

"Hey, Austin," everyone said in unison.

"Hi, honey." My mother acknowledged me as well.

88

"Hi, Mom," I said.

There was a large round table, and on the table was a laptop with a file that had my name on it. There were three people who sat across from me. One was a woman, and the other two were men. Mr. Tate sat next to me on the right, and Doctor Jerry sat next to me on the left. Doctor Jerry was wearing a blue button shirt with black dress slacks. My mom sat in the corner of the small room that was next to the mental health board members. The two men who sat across from me wore average looking clothing, no suits or ties, and the one on the left in front of me was wearing overalls. He was also wearing a white plain t-shirt, and he had white hair and peach colored skin. His nose was large, and his eyes were beady. He looked to be in his forties or fifties. The man to my left was also white, and he wore a plain black t-shirt. He had a smaller nose than the man to my left. The man to my right had brown hair and appeared to be in his late thirties. The woman who sat in the middle had on a gray dress. She was the only one dressed up nice. Her buttons were silver, and her hair was black. My mom sat in the corner with her black bag and her notebook. My mom had on a silver sparkling shirt, and it had a butterfly on it. My mom's hair looked beautiful, and she had a silver hair pen in her hair.

"Okay, the sole purpose for this hearing is to determine if Austin Bower needs to be placed in a psychiatric hospital for his condition and his mental health state of mind," Doctor Jerry said.

There was a microphone in front of me on the table.

"How do you feel about this, Mr. Tate?"

"Well, I believe with my professional opinion that sending Austin to the hospital is in his best interest," Mr. Tate said.

"How does your client feel about this?"

"He stated he believes he is unsafe to the community and to himself right now," Mr Tate said.

"Mr. Bower, is this true?" Dr. Jerry began to probe the question.

"Yes," I said. I leaned into the microphone to speak.

"Do we have a yes from the board members?"

"Yes," the man on the left said.

"Yes," the woman in the middle said.

"Yes," the man on the right said.

"Okay, we have our verdict," Dr. Jerry said.

I stood up and gave my mother a brief hug, and soon after Mr. Tate escorted me back to the unit.

Chapter 8 Building Ten

The Lincoln Regional Center in Lincoln, Nebraska places those who are civilly commited at risk for violence by mixing criminally committed patients with the civilly committed patients.

F riday had come around, and I was in my room reading a book that I found in the library. The book was based on the United States Constitution and the amendments for the people. It included the first ten amendments, which were otherwise known as the Bill of Rights. I read through the book over the week, and I enjoyed what the Constitution had to offer. It spoke on laws that had also been ratified during Lincoln's term in regard to the slave days. I felt like a slave, and I knew what I was feeling wasn't right. I felt confined and locked up. I felt withdrawn from everything and everyone. I was laying in bed just finishing the last few pages that the book had to offer. I walked out of my room, and I saw six other patients walking around the unit. Two were female and four were male patients. Misty was one of the patients walking, and Chris was walking too. The techs on duty were Kelly, Jim, and some girl that I hadn't seen before. She had black hair, pale skin, a long nose, and blue eyes. She was pretty, I thought. I walked further out of my room to get a closer look at her.

"Austin," Jim said.

"Ya."

"The nurse needs you at the medication window," he said.

"Okay."

I walked to the nurse's window, and it was a new nurse I hadn't seen before.

"Hello Austin, I am Christi," she said.

"Hi Christi," I said.

I didn't smile.

"Here are your medications, and here is some water," she said.

"The doctor put you on a new pill," she said.

"What is it?"

"It looks like he put you on Prozac," she said.

"I can't take Prozac," I said. "I'm allergic to it."

"Well it looks like he wants you on it," she said.

"What is going on?"

"First it was depikote, and now it is Prozac," I said. "Don't you people understand that I am allergic to certain medications?" I said.

"Well Austin....dear, you have to take them," she said.

"I can't. It gives me allergic reactions," I said.

"Well then it will just be a refusal," she said.

"Then I refuse!"

"Okay," she said. "I will be sure to tell the doctor," she said.

She said it like it was an open threat.

"Austin, are you going to take your meds or not?"

"I will take the other two, but I won't take the Prozac," I said.

"Okay, that is your choice, but keep in mind if you don't take them, we can put you in full beds for not being medication compliant," she said.

"I don't care. I have a right to refuse medication, and there is nothing that you can do about it," I said.

"Oh, yes there is," she said. "Hey Kelly," she yelled. "Kelly, would you come over here please?"

"Okay, I will take my medication," I said.

"That's a good boy, and don't try to fight it, or it will get worse," she said. "Do your best to accept what is happening."

She sounded evil when I heard her say that to me. I thought she was the devil's sister. I took the Prozac, and I swallowed it with the water she gave me.

"Austin, we can't have you eat breakfast yet," Kelly said.

Kelly came closer.

"You have a lab draw today," he said. "We need you to not eat anything until after your lab draw."

Kelly was wearing a black dress shirt and a pair of blue jeans. He was also wearing a pair of Jordan tennis shoes. They had the jump man on the side, and it read twenty-three on the front of his shoe. They were black and red. I was bothered by the fact that I couldn't eat, however the food was nasty, so I didn't really care. Either way it sucked, and I hated the place that I was in. The lab tech came on the floor. She had on a white lab coat with Loony Tunes characters on her lab pants.

"You must be Austin," she said.

"Yes," I said.

"Let's get your lab work done," she said.

She had spunk to her voice. She had blond hair, and she was short and skinny.

"What's your name?"

"I'm Sue," she said. "Or otherwise known as the vampire."

She had a lab kit with her, and it was a see through container. She pulled out some empty vials and needles that were designed to go into the vials. She had on blue latex gloves, and she pulled out rubbing alcohol packets. She tore the packets open, and you could smell the alcohol automatically. She rubbed the alcohol on my right arm, and then she took the needle and she stuck me. I watched as the blood flowed out into the vile. Sue then took the first vile, and she placed it into the container. She followed up by putting the smaller vial into the needle wedge. When she was all done, she placed names on all the vials, and then she set them in a unique order in the clear container. She then put medical tape and a cotton ball on my arm for a bandage.

"Thanks Austin, that's all I need," she said.

I walked away, and I got ready for breakfast. The techs had set my tray to the side. I then sat down, and I was given my tray. It was fifteen minutes until nine in the morning. After I was given my tray, I sat down to eat my breakfast. The food was cold and stale. I felt like not even eating. I had to though, for survival. I had to eat this nasty food, whether I wanted to or not. This food was disgusting, but I ate it anyway. I was angry at the world right now, and I was on edge and paranoid. I was seated at the dining room table just to be there. Just so I could pass time. I had been in the crisis center for over two weeks now, and I hated it. I hated the feeling of it, and I couldn't stand it or the people. I just didn't want to be here anymore.

"Austin," Kelly said.

"Ya."

"They want you at the front of the building, so we need you to pack your belongings," he said.

"I'm leaving?"

"You're leaving," he said.

I went to my room, and the tech handed me a plastic bag, and I began to pack my belongings. I was in a rush, and I had no idea where I was going to next. I had my belongings in one large plastic bag, and I was ready to roll. A guard in a brown uniform came up to me with full body chains.

"Bower," he said.

He looked at me without a smile. He had brown hair and a strong build.

"We will be taking you to the state hospital," he said.

"Okay."

"Let's get these chains on you," he said.

I began to allow him to shackle me. He had a black box with him too. I was afraid of where I was going. I had never been to the state hospital before. The guard had me all chained up, and he carried my belongings for me. We went through the doors the same way we came. It was just the opposite way. I was led down the elevator, and then into a county vehicle. I had to be careful clearing my step because the chains hugged my ankles. I was seated in the middle of the van. The sun was out, and it was a little cloudy. It looked like it just rained outside too. The guard buckled my seat belt for me. Then he headed to the driver side. He had a funny name, and it was one that I couldn't pronounce. He began to drive, and the guard slowly pulled out of the driveway. We went through all the stop lights, and we had passed through all the city streets. We went through downtown, and we took Rosa Parks Boulevard. We headed down to Folson Road and passed by some train tracks. I watched as I came into the area. There were trees everywhere, and the guard drove up the paved road. The road had led to large buildings that looked like something from the past. The buildings looked old and worn out. I thought they needed remodeling for sure. The guard began looking for the area of where I was supposed to be. The closer he got to the buildings, the more detail of them I could see. They looked even older up close than they did from a distance. The trees looked dried up and withered. I sat in the van feeling uncomfortable in the cuffs that I was in. I looked through the window of the van, and I saw things from a different view. The guard pulled to a complete stop, and he got on to his radio to speak a few words. He then wrote something down on a piece of paper, which was connected to his clipboard.

"Okay, Austin, this is it," he said.

I noticed that this was the first time the guard called

me by my first name. It would probably be the last time too, I thought. I waited for him to open the door and escort me out. As he opened the door, he then stood back to give me space, so I could get out on my own. I slowly stood up, and I stepped down meeting the ground. Once on the ground the guard shut the door, and then he led the way, and I followed. He led me into a building that had large windows in the front. There were shriveled up bushes in the front of the building. The guard pressed a button so we could be let into the building. We both waited patiently to be let in. After standing outside for a few minutes, an older white lady came to the door and opened the door for us. The guard didn't talk much. He said a few words here and there, but that was about it. I think he kept it that way on purpose. The guard led me into the building, and after I was led in, the white lady went around to the back of the front desk. The guard walked up to the counter, and he checked me in. The guard filled out a few things of paperwork and signed his name as well. I stood right next to him as he filled out the paperwork. The lobby to the building ten waiting room had both black and brown chairs in it. It also had a long brown table that seemed to be low to the ground. The counter that the guard was at had a long counter top and a cup with pens in it. Near the counter was a door, and that door led to a few back rooms, including the room behind the counter. Once he was finished, the guard then removed my chains.

After that the guard took the exit, and he carried all the chains with him too, even dragging some of them on the floor. I was left alone with the Lincoln Regional Center staff. There were two techs and a nurse present waiting for me, and a lady that was from admissions wanted to take my photo. She asked me to stand next to the white wall, and I was unchained. I wore a plain white t-shirt and a pair of Levi blue jeans. I stood against the wall, and the lady took my picture. The lady had blond hair, and she looked to be middle aged. She wasn't ugly by any means, and she had a very pretty smile to her. She wore a white sweater and a pair of blue jeans. Her shoes were silver and white. The two techs waiting for me to do intake were both white. One of them was tall and large, and the other one was short and fat. The tall tech had on Jordan boots, and they were black and silver. He also painted his fingernails black, and his entire outfit was black as well. I thought of him to be in some type of goth cult or something. The shorter one had on a Nike sweater and a pair of blue jeans with white running shoes. The nurse was white with blond hair, and she had large breasts. She was thin and appeared to work out on a regular basis. She had on black slacks and a white lab coat, and under her lab coat was a yellow shirt. There were many hallways to the first floor, and there were many rooms too. The doors were all made of wood, and they looked heavy and large. The handles to the doors were a grayish color.

99

"Hi Austin, I am Josh and I will be your assigned tech today," Josh said.

"Okay," I said.

"Hi Austin, I am Dan," Dan said.

"Nice to meet you both," I said.

"Hello Austin, I will be your assigned nurse, and my name is Tammra," Tammra said.

"Hi Tammra, it's nice to meet you."

My photo was taken by the long white hallway wall, and from there Dan and Josh escorted me to an elevator that would lead me to my unit. I waited for Dan to use his key for us to enter the elevator. You couldn't get on or off the elevator without a key. Once he was finished, I entered the elevator. The elevator smelled bad, like something was dying.

"What is that smell?"

I was covering my nose with my shirt.

"That's just the plumbing," Josh said. "Something is wrong with it."

"It smells terrible," I said.

The elevator doors opened, and I entered the unit, and I noticed seven people walking around. Some were old and some were young. There was a young man with glasses and red hair who was talking to another person, who appeared to be a patient. The patient that he was talking to looked black and had curly hair. I saw another patient in a wheelchair, and his feet looked swollen, like two balloons. The patient in the wheelchair seemed to be talking louder than normal. I then saw another patient whose hand had a medical bandage on it. He was black and had a thin face and was also skinny. The unit was noisy and seemed to be out of control. I walked up the unit hallway, and I saw eight other patients in a large room. These patients looked to be mostly white, and only a few were black. They were all playing a board game of sorts. Possible Monopoly? I wasn't sure.

"Austin," Josh said.

"Ya."

"I will be showing you where your room is," he said.

"Okay."

Josh led me to a nearby room down the hallway.

"This is where you will be staying," he said. "Your roommate's name is Mike."

"Okay, thank you," I said.

"You bet. Oh, and we will be doing your paperwork together later today," he said.

"Okay, what kind of paperwork?"

"Just admissions stuff."

"Okay, thank you."

"You are very welcome."

Josh walked away, and I was left in my room to myself. I sat on my bed, and I began to relax. I hated the ride up here, I thought, and those chains were the worst. I laid on my bed for about twenty minutes, and then Dan came by.

"Knock, knock," Dan said. "Here are your belongings."

He was holding a large plastic bag in his hand.

"We went through your belongings, and we had to take away your shoe strings," Dan said. "Which by the way, we will need your strings out of those shoes too," he said.

"But I want to keep my shoe strings," I said.

"Well, you can't. I am sorry, but those are the rules here."

"Bullshit, I want to keep my shoe strings," I said.

"Well either you give me your shoe strings, or I bring in more staff, and we will take them from you," he said.

"Is that a threat?"

I was standing up now.

"No, that's just policy," he said. "The choice is your own."

"Well, I don't want to give them up," I said.

"Okay, suit yourself," he said.

The tech got on his radio, and he began to contact other staff claiming I was being uncooperative. Staff came flooding into my room by the numbers.

"He won't give up his shoe strings," Dan said.

"Okay, hold him down," Tammra said.

The nurse showed her true colors right then and there I thought.

"Hold him down," Dan said.

Josh came in, and four other techs came in after him. Then they grabbed me by my arms and my legs as I began to resist.

"Get the restraints!"

I was on my bed squirming to get the staff off of me. I wasn't putting up a big fight, but I was resisting. The techs held me down, and then things got worse. One of the techs placed his knee on my throat, and at this point, I realized they had done this before. His knee was applying so much pressure to my throat, and I could hardly breathe.

"You will give us the shoe strings, Austin, whether you want to or not," Dan said.

"Okay, you can have them," I said.

"What are we going to do?"

"He is going to full beds," Tammra said. "I will get his shot ready."

"Shot, what fucking shot! I don't want a fucking shot," I said.

"Do you have the restraints?"

"Yes, they are coming," Dan said.

"I just heard them call it on the radio," he said.

I was squirming and moving around while they had me in their grasp. They brought the restraints and placed them on me, one by one. I could feel them as they lifted each arm at a time. They would strap me in these leather restraints, and then have a special key to lock them. I was still on the bed while they were fixing the restraints on me. It felt abnormal. It felt weird, and I was scared. They removed my shoes off of my feet, and I felt them tugging to remove them. Thoughts of going to prison entered my mind. The memories of my past entered my thoughts. After they had the restraints on me, they moved me from one section of the unit to another.

"Can you walk, Austin?"

"Yes, I can walk," I said.

They lifted me up and I began to walk to the full bedroom. They led me down the hallway, and we passed the staff desk.

"Go to your rooms," Dan said.

Other patients were watching as I was being shuffled along to my next destination. Once the staff had me

104

there, they laid me on a bed mat, and it had straps on it. They brought me to the center of it, and one by one they used a key to untie my restraints. Then they placed my limbs into the restraints, one by one. The nurse then came into the full bedroom.

"Are you ready for your shot?"

"No, I don't want a shot," I cried.

"Well, you should have thought about that before you decided not to give up your shoe strings," she said.

"Okay, let's give him the shot."

"No, I don't want it," I said.

I was squirming.

"Okay, hold him down," she said.

Two techs came to hold me down; one of them was Josh.

"I'm sorry, Austin," Josh said.

"Don't apologize to him," Tammra said. "Hold him down and do your job."

"No, I don't want the shot!Get your hands off of me!"

"Austin, calm down," Josh said.

"Please Austin, you need to stop fighting it," he said.

"No, I don't want it! No stop, I don't want it!"

Tammra began to place the needle against my arm, and she forced the shot into my skin.

"Hold still," she said.

"No, I don't want it!"

I was screaming as loud as I could.

"No!...No!....No!"

My voice was going out from yelling, and my throat felt raspy.

"All done. You see, that wasn't so bad," she said. "Now go to sleep, and rest there for a while."

She sounded like a demon from Satan. I feared her, and I had a good reason to. I laid on the full bed restraint table crying. Tears were flowing down my face. I was so upset. The room was small, and there was a window on the left side of the room. One tech remained outside the room at all times. The techs would change places every thirty minutes, and while being outside the room, they would chart. They kept a clipboard and charted all of my movements. They charted my words, and they charted me just being there.

"My restraints are too tight," I said.

"I feel like they are cutting off my circulation."

The tech had no response at all. She said nothing, and all she did was write what she heard.

"I want up! Please, let me up!"

Nothing and no one came to my rescue. I was in pain emotionally, and I was drained spiritually. I felt

106

ignored and neglected. The nurse came back into the room.

"Austin, if you don't stop yelling, your time will start all over," she said.

"Go fuck yourself!"

"That's it, your time has started over," she said.

I laid there for over an hour. I wanted to be let up, but I had no support. I was angry, but I knew now that I had to stay calm if I wanted to make it out of this. So I did, and I waited it out. I remained calm, and I eventually fell into a deep sleep.

Chapter 9 Lincoln Regional Center

Individuals with Autism Spectrum Disorder, (ASD) interact with others differently. They often appear to have difficulty understanding and expressing emotion, and may express attachment in a different manner.

I realized that I wouldn't make it far in the process of things if I continued to go back and forth from the full bedroom to the isolation room. I just knew that this would go against me in the larger deal of things. I was afraid to go to prison, and I wasn't ready for it either. I would do anything to slow the process down if I could. I couldn't stand the thought of being put in such a place. I often had racing thoughts about it, and I was unsure of my future. I had on a green Mountain Dew baseball cap, and a pair of blue jeans, brought in by my mother. Life was hectic and noisy on the unit that I was on. I met this red head kid after I got out of full bed restraints.

"Yo, what's up man?"

"My name is Pete, what's your name, dog?"

"Well, I'm not a dog," I said.

"Oh, no I was just clowning around. "But, seriously, what's your name?"

"I'm Austin," I said.

"Yo, that's cool," he said.

He seemed to be high on drugs or something. He had freckles on his face and red hair on his head. He also wore gold framed glasses. He had on brown khaki pants and a brown khaki shirt.

"I do what I do, and how 'bout you?" he said.

"Cause I ain't no punk, and I got nice shoes," he was rapping now.

"I love my music, and don't you abuse it."

"Fuck all you haters, and all you skaters."

"Well I used to skate, so that made no sense," he said.

I kept listening to his rap songs, and they annoyed me, so I walked away. I thought he had wishful thinking if he wanted to become a rap artist. I felt uncomfortable around him, and I just didn't see anything good coming about hanging around him. I walked down the hallway and went into my bedroom to lay down. I laid there for a long time, and I eventually just fell asleep. I was tired of everything. I was tired of taking orders and having to listen to other people tell me what to do or how it was going to be. It got old after a while, and it wasn't getting any better. I slept all the way until it was time for chow. I woke up ten minutes before dinner was being served. I walked into the hallway and into the large dining room that was meant for meals, breakfast,

lunch, and dinner. I wondered if the food here was
better than the food in the county. Everyone was
lining up in single file, one person at a time, and I
lined up. I was second in line, and I waited behind
this black guy. He had an afro, and he was tall and
large. His face was thick, and his eyes were brown. I
didn't know his name, and I never asked him either.
There were about eighteen other people behind me in
line. Some were skinny and some were fat. I waited
until they called dinner.

"Tonight you are having spaghetti," Kendra said.

She was black and had curly black hair. Her legs
were thick, and she had a strong upper build to her
body. She wore a green shirt and blue jeans. She had
a badge around her neck.

"*DHHS, Kendra,*" the badge read, and her photo was
underneath her name.

She was wearing white and purple shoes. I thought
she was attractive for a black women. She had a gap
in between her teeth, and that made her more
attractive. Her lips were full, and she had high cheek
bones. She began to walk in front of me. Her hips
would swing in motion, and it almost looked like she
was dancing. She had a graceful walk to her, and she
reminded me of my girlfriend. She was black and
had thick hips like Kendra. I remember the first day
that I met Sarah. I spoke to her outside of an
apartment complex in Lincoln, Nebraska. It was an

110

unhealthy relationship for sure. She often threatened me and hit me if I didn't do what she wanted. I was taught not to hit women back. So when Sarah hit me I would just take it, and I thought it was normal. I wouldn't hit her back, even if it meant getting her off of me in that moment. Kendra looked an awful lot like Sarah. This made it harder for me to work with her as a patient.

"You must be Austin. Are you feeling better?"

Kendra approached me while I was in line.

Her voice was attractive, and she had a soft spoken, low tone voice for a women. Her eyes were deceptive, and she was wearing blue eyeliner makeup.

"Yes, I am okay," I said.

"Good," she said. "I am happy to hear it."

The dining room had white walls and the tables were round. The room had windows that gazed onto the outside world. I looked the food over, and I began to eat my spaghetti, and it tasted better than the county food. I enjoyed it, and it was hotter than the county food too. I guess the state hospital made sure their food was hot. It was high in carbs, nevertheless it was hot. I finished my meal, and then I put my dish in a big bin. The staff counted the silver wear after we finished eating. I assumed they did this every meal. The day went by with meaningless conversation. I hadn't had a shower yet, but I felt like

111

I needed one. It was seven o'clock in the evening, and I wanted to shower before my medication time. I went to the staff desk, and I saw Kendra standing at the counter.

"Kendra?"

I waited for her to respond.

"Yes, how can I help you, Austin?"

"Can I please have a towel and a wash cloth?"

"Sure," she said. "Do you need any shampoo and conditioner?"

"Yes, please," I said.

"Okay, hold these while I get your shampoo and your conditioner," she said.

She handed me the towel and the wash cloth. I waited patiently for her. She stood with her back to me. The shampoo and the conditioner were both in a bucket on the ground in bottles.

"Do you want your shampoo, and conditioner in a cup?"

"Yes please," I said.

She slowly stood up, and she handed me my hygiene supplies. I then went to the shower room, which was a few doors down from my bedroom. Kendra followed me to unlock the shower door. She smiled at me in the process of doing so.

"Have a nice shower," she said.

"Okay, thank you," I replied.

I went to take my shower, and I felt like I was in slow motion. I put my head under the water, and it was warm. The water was dripping down my neck, and I began to cry. I wept for a while, and then a knock came at the door.

"Hurry up in there, I need to shower too!"

"Okay, I'll be right out," I said.

The water was still running, and I had no intention of shutting it off right away. I showered for five more minutes, and then I shut the water off. I dried myself off, and then I got myself dressed. From there I headed to my room, and I went to my room until medication time. At eight o'clock I came out, and I went to the med window. It was a different nurse than the one before. This nurse seemed to be more polite and less conniving than Tammra. I took my medication, and then I headed off to bed. Over the weekend it was the same routine, but the only difference was the food because the food was on a four week cycle. Plus nothing happened on the weekend. It was an off day for the practicing psychiatric staff. I continued to take my medications and my showers. It was noisy, nevertheless I really didn't have a choice but to be here. Monday came, and it was a new day. I was scheduled for court, and that meant getting out of the hospital for a few hours, or so I thought until I was told otherwise.

"Austin, they canceled your court for today," Josh said.

"Do you know when I will have it next?"

"I couldn't tell ya, bud," Josh said.

Josh had on a red t-shirt and a pair of blue jeans. I watched as he walked away. Josh had a clipboard in his hands, so I figured he was making rounds doing his checks. I wanted court to be done with, and I wanted the charges to be dropped. Nevertheless, I realized that wouldn't happen. I paced the hallway back and forth until things began to pick up for activities. I learned that they had groups and yard activities. The hospital even had its own canteen area, where they cooked french fries, burgers, and so many other things. The hospital staff allowed me to keep thirty dollars on my person. So I was allowed to use that money for food and drinks at the canteen. I was still on the unit when they called for yard. The techs on the floor were Josh, Dan, Kevin, Michael, Stacy, and Lorance.

"Yard!"

Everyone who wanted to go began to line up for yard. I got in line as well, and some lined up by the elevator, and others lined up near the stairs.

"I'm going," Pete said.

"Me too," I said.

"Austin, you can't go to yard," Dan said.

"Why not?"

"Because you are on assault precautions," Dan said.

"For what?"

"You know why," he said.

"No, I don't know. I want you to tell me," I said.

"You know why," he said.

"No, I don't. I honestly don't know why," I said.

"Ask Josh; he would be glad to tell you," Dan said.

I left out of line in search for Josh, and I began looking for him down the hallway and near my room. I had no luck finding him at all. So I decided just to go to my room and lay down. I laid there for about an hour, and I had my face in the pillow.

"Austin," Lorance said.

My face was still in the pillow.

"What?"

My voice was muffled.

"The team wants to meet with you," Lorance said.

I was seated up now with my arm resting on the bed. The mattress was hard and unpleasant to lay on.

"Okay...what does that mean?"

"They want to review your status," he said.

I rose up and followed Lorance into the hallway, and he led me down towards a conference room into the other hallway. There were two hallways on this unit. One to the left, and one to the right. I walked up to the door, and there were three people seated in a large room, and the room had a long wooden table. There was a woman along with two men. They had paper in their hands and on the desk, and one of them had a briefcase.

"Hello, Austin," the woman said. "I am Doctor Moore."

She had red hair and brown eyes, and her eyes were beady.

"I am your psychologist assigned to your case, Austin," Dr. Moore said. "Please take a seat."

I went to sit down, and I pulled out a chair. The other two men were quiet. One appeared to be Asian, and the other looked to be Persian.

"Austin, we are meeting with you today in regards to your status," she said. "You are currently on assault precautions. How are you feeling?"

"I'm okay," I said.

"You don't feel like hurting any one?"

"No, I don't," I said.

"Okay.... well over the weekend you did a pretty good job of staying out of trouble. So we will place you on twenty-four hour motivational level," she said.

"What's that?"

"Well, it's a level that only allows you to go to yard and groups, however you can't go to canteen," she said.

Doctor Moore was soft spoken, and it almost seemed like she whispered when she spoke.

"Please sign this form here, stating that you agree with the decision," she said.

She handed me a pen, and I signed my name on the form.

"Okay, thank you, Austin," she said.

"You're welcome," I said.

I began to exit the room. The two other men never even said a word. I thought that was odd. I sort of felt ignored by the both of them. As I went into the hallway, a rush of noise entered the unit. Patients were returning from their yard activities. I still hadn't gone to yard since my arrival. I wondered if they had a basketball court. The day went by yet again, with more meaningless talk of sports and celebrities. All in all it was pretty meaningless. No educational practice and no types of skill building for higher learning. It was almost as if they wanted to keep me stupid or something of that nature. The night went by with the same routine, and I took my medication and decided to call it a night. Tuesday came around, and this time I took a shower in the morning, instead of during the night. I washed up and cleaned myself off. I then brushed my teeth and I got dressed into the outfit my mother had brought me. I had a pair of shorts, a white t-shirt, and a pair of Nike shower shoes. I had shower shoes on my feet to prevent me from getting athlete's foot.

"Yard!"

This time I would be able to out, I thought, and I was thankful for that too. I lined up in file, and only six other people were in line with me. Pete didn't line up today. In a way I was kind of happy about Pete not going to yard with us. I thought that he was annoying and loud. I also thought he was stupid. He followed suit on what the government wanted him to do, taking any kind of medication they gave him to stay doped up. I was one to talk, though, because I kind of fell into the same mix, and it wasn't by choice. I was threatened with full beds and isolation if I didn't take the medication given to me. So maybe I was the stupid one, and he was the smart one. That was the conclusion that I came to. I felt stupid as it was because I followed Hawkboy and his unrealistic guidance. I listened to a criminal to be where I was. However, I had no idea he was a criminal. He told me that we were going to a party to drink and meet women. He never told me that we would rob someone. I must have been the stupid one, I thought.

118

Josh went up to the door and unlocked it, and we were headed to yard. I noticed that Dan wasn't working today, and that made me a little happy. Nevertheless he would be back, but for now I enjoyed my peace of mind that he wasn't here. Josh led us down two flights of stairs and three doors to get to the yard that we were going to. He took his badge and swiped it across the door, and the door opened.

"Wow, it's still nice out," Josh said. "I thought that it was supposed to rain today."

"Well, I am thankful it didn't," I said.

I grabbed the first basketball that I could find, and I began shooting baskets. I would dribble and spin, duck and jump, and I could do it all.

"Come on, Josh," I said.

"No, I better not."

"Why, am I too good for you or something?"

"No, I just better not," he said.

"Okay," I said.

I continued shooting baskets, and I felt free when I did. I felt so alive, and it was amazing, and I loved the rush that it gave me. I kept shooting baskets until Josh told me and the group that yard time was over. The yard door was big and red. In the yard there was a patio and a large cement wall that blocked anyone from getting in or getting out. After Josh called for yard to be over, we as a group lined up in single file. We returned to the unit, as a group, the same way that we came out. When I returned a doctor was waiting on me to do an evaluation, and I acknowledged her presence.

"Hi, are you Austin?"

"Yes, I am Austin," I said.

"Can you please come with me to do your evaluation?"

"Ya, sure."

The doctor was very pretty, and she had brown hair and brown skin. She was thin and had thick legs. For her outfit she had on a red dress and high heels. Her dress only came down to her knees, and she looked intelligent. I knew she was smart—she had to be to be a doctor. She led me into a room, and no one else followed. The room had white walls and a small table. In front of the table were two chairs, and the light seemed to be off, but it wasn't.

"So, Austin, my name is Doctor Luda," she said. "I will be doing your evaluation for court."

"Okay, let's get started," I said.

Doctor Luda smiled at me, and I saw her teeth were perfectly even. Doctor Luda pulled out a large folder that was made out of leather. She began to ask me a series of questions that constituted memory. She asked me to repeat numbers, letters, and words in the order that she gave. I did as she asked, and after words she moved me along to another project. This time she used pictures, and she had me point at what was missing in the photograph that she provided. Then she moved along to black spots, where she asked me what I thought the spots represented. She also asked me what I saw in the black spots in my own opinion. I told her my opinion of what I saw, and how I saw it. The testing took about an hour to two hours. When she finished the testing, she congratulated me for doing my best, and that she felt confident in the results. When we were done I went back to my room, and I laid down thinking of how I wish this wasn't my life right now. Nevertheless, it was my life for right now, and all that I could do was accept it for what it was in the moment. I laid in bed, and I skipped lunch. I had no desire to eat right now.

"Lunchtime, Austin," Stacy said.

She popped her head into my room.

"I'm not hungry right now," I said.

"Are you sure?"

"Yes, I am sure," I said.

"Okey, dokey," she said.

She began to walk away. I laid on my bed avoiding groups and other activities just because I felt so low. The day carried on into the night, and I watched the sun slowly fade until the moon took over. It was as if they were holding the balance of all humanity in their hands, and the moon was taking over the night shift. I came out of my room at about seven o'clock, and I walked the hallway up and down. I skipped both lunch and dinner because I wasn't very hungry for many reasons.

"Austin, you have a visitor," Kendra said.

She smiled when she spoke.

"Are you ready?"

"Yes," I said.

"Kendra to one hundred, is it clear to send one to visiting?"

"You're clear," the voice said.

"Austin, let's get you to your visit," she said.

Kendra unlocked the door and began to escort me down to the canteen, which is where visiting is held.

"So who is coming to see you?"

"My mom, probably," I said.

We were alone as she was walking me down the flight of stairs. There was no one in the hallway.

"Well, I hope that you have a good visit," she said.

"Thanks," I said.

I continued down the stairs, and she led the way.

When we arrived my mom had on a baseball cap, and she brought in some Burger King from the nearby burger joint. She had the burger already laid out, and along with it were french fries.

"Hey Mom!"

I gave my mom a big hug.

"How are you doing?"

I sat down, and Kendra was staring at me from the other side of the room.

"Um.... I'm okay," I said.

"Are you sure?"

"Ya," I said.

I began to cry because I was afraid to go to prison.

"What's wrong, honey?"

"Nothing Mom, I'll be okay," I said.

The tears were falling down my face like a waterfall.

"Here, give me a hug," she said.

"Okay."

I was afraid to go to prison, and I was unsure if I would be going there or not.

"Mom, I am afraid," I said.

"Of what, honey?"

"I'm afraid that I will go to prison," I said.

"It will be okay, just give it over to God," she said.

"And do what, Mom? Do what with God?"

"Pray," she said.

"Pray? You want me to pray?"

"Yes, honey, pray," she said.

I began to agree with her.

"Okay, Mom, I will pray," I said.

We were both seated now. The visit took my mind off of everything else. It was as if it wasn't real. It was like time slowed down, and my mother and I were in a warm hole of time. The visit went by with talk of family and me eating my french fries and burger. After the visit I gave my mother a hug, and we both separated. I was back on the unit, and I took my medications from the nurse on duty. Then right after taking my meds, I went to bed.

Every day seemed the same at the Lincoln Regional Center; nothing else was new. It was noisy and busy. The patients were like grown children. They were all lost souls, especially Pete. That soul was lost for sure. I spent four long months in this forsaken hospital, and every day I was pulling my hair out wanting to leave, and I had no desire to stay. The sad thing about it is the fact that I think they wanted to keep me there. Crazy to think such an idea, but I believed it. Some of these staff were ill minded. Not all of them, though, because I felt that Josh and

Kendra were pretty good people. It seemed to be the other batch, and that is not a fallacy by any measure. So I continued to go to the awful groups that were given to me, and they were led by horrible group leaders. I just couldn't believe that they couldn't find a sense of control for these crazy patients. They were loud, and obnoxious, and overwhelming to live around. I had a roommate, yet he never spoke to me. He often laid on his bed like I did and pretended to be oblivious to everything that was happening. The weekend went by, and Monday came around. I was in my room when I got the news.

"Austin, pack your belongings," Dan said.

He sounded a little happy too. So I gathered my belongings, and I was escorted down the elevator, and awaiting me was the guard in the brown uniform.

Chapter 10 Court Appearance

Today the majority of Psychiatric hospital beds in America are court ordered beds. Meaning the criminal system has become the new mental health system in America. Leaving those individuals who truly have mental health needs unnoticed, and ignored.

I walked in the courtroom wearing the full body chain restraints, provided by the county. I was escorted by the county bailiff. The courtroom had polished wood and beautiful green chairs. The chairs were wooden with green padding. There was a large L shaped table and microphones built into the table. I saw a small black box, and it had wires hooked to it. The box was facing a large white screen, and I assumed the courts used this equipment for trials. The bailiff was wearing a silver badge, and he had a set of keys. There was a lady seated at the bottom of the pulpit. At the top of the pulpit was a rather large leather chair, and the lady had a keyboard in front of her.

"Okay, Bower, take a seat right here," the bailiff said.

I noticed that my attorney hadn't shown up yet, and I really wanted to talk with him. The judge wasn't quite in yet, and I didn't know if this was a good thing or a bad thing. I saw a motion in the corner of my eye. Mac had shown up after all, and he had a black suitcase with him. Mac was wearing a gray suit and a red tie, and his hair was combed rather than messy. His shoes were black wing toe dress shoes. Mac came and sat beside me in the empty chair.

"Austin," Mac whispered, "we will not be doing your plea today," he said.

"Okay, what does that mean?"

"It means this is a court appearance," he said.

I became a little nervous and anxious, and I didn't know what all of this meant because it was my first time ever in this situation. I had never been to court like this before. I was afraid of what would happen, and prison entered my mind. I knew I wouldn't make it in prison.

"Can I speak with my client alone?"

"Sure," the bailiff said.

"Here, come with me, Austin," Mac said.

I followed Mac a short distance, and he led me into a small waiting room near the court entrance. I sat down in a plastic chair while Mac stood over me.

"Austin, I want you to know Hawkboy took a plea bargain today for a lesser charge," Mac said.

"I didn't take a plea bargain yet," I said.

"I know," Mac said. "Do you want to take one?"

"What's the bargain?"

"A class three felony," Mac said.

"A class three?"

"Yes," Mac said.

"What's that carry up to?"

"It's a one to twenty," Mac said.
"So I can get up to twenty years?"

"It's better than the fifty that you were facing," he said.

"That's true. Okay."

"Okay?" Mac hesitated.

"Ya, let's do it," I said.

"Okay," Mac said.

I walked back to my seat while dragging along with me the burden of the chains. I took my seat in my original spot. I sat there not knowing what was going to happen.

"All rise for the honorable Judge Chaos," the Court Clerk said.

I rose and so did Mac and the county bailiff. The District Attorney was already standing, and she had blond hair and fair skin. She was wearing a black dress with black high heels. The District Attorney had a crossed eye, and it made her look ugly. She was tall, and chubby, and her name was Jerkenson. The judge came into the courtroom, and he was tall with white hair, and he had a beard. He was wearing a black robe that went over his suit. His robe made it look like he was getting a haircut. His robe looked cheap and cheesy.

"This is the court appearance for the defendant Mr. Bower," Chaos said.

"State your name for the record, and whom is representing Mr. Bower," Chaos said.

"Kevin Mac," Mac said.

"State your name for the record," Chaos said.

"District Attorney Jerkenson," Jerkenson said.

"State who you are representing, in the case of the defendant," Chaos said.

"Austin Bower," Mac said.

"Mr. Bower, state your name for the record," Chaos said.

"Hello, I am Austin Bower," I said.

"Austin, do you wish for Kevin Mac to represent you?"

"Yes," I said.

"Well, your honor," Mac said, "if I may."

"You may," Chaos said.

"My client needs a further evaluation," Mac said.

"Your wish is denied," Chaos said.

"We are not going to spend taxpayer money for a criminal to relax in our state hospital. He has already spent four months undergoing an evaluation," Chaos said.

"We need more time," Mac said.

"I'm sending this case to district court," Chaos said. "Bail set at five hundred thousand, court dismissed."

Chapter 11 The County Jail

I was back in the Lincoln County Correctional Facility. I was housed in the special needs unit this time. I lived on the upper teir, and my cell viewed the entire unit, even the shower. I was in the upper right hand corner of the unit. The food sucked as it always did. I couldn't get used to it, and I didn't know how half the population ate it. There were meals that I just wouldn't touch because it looked unsafe to. The special needs unit split their time in half with the protective custody unit. So other inmates in general population often thought I was a P.C. inmate, which I wasn't, but I could see how they could confuse me with someone who was. I mean it was the same unit after all. I had very little friends in the county jail, and I sort of liked it that way. The friends that I did have were no friends at all. I only did business with them because it was means for survival, and I wanted to survive. One of my so-called friends was the housing porter. So he got extra goodies for doing his job, and sometimes I even received soda, which soda pop was not something that was given out freely. This friend of mine would pour soda in a cup for me if I bought him something that he couldn't afford on the canteen list.

"So Jack, can I get some soda from you tonight?"

"Ya, that's cool," he said.

"Just make sure you have a Kit Kat bar for me this Monday," he said.

"Alright."

I was playing cards at the table with Jack, Mitch, and Kramer. We were playing four man spades, and I was on Jack's team. Jack had a tattoo of a ghost with a needle shooting his arm up with dope. Matter of fact, the word 'dope' was spelled out on his arm. He also had a tattoo underneath his eye, and under his eye was a tear drop.

"So, what are you bidding, Austin?"

"I'm bidding three," I said.

"Okay, I am bidding four," he said.

"So lets go seven," I said.

"Na, lets go eight," Jack said.

"Um...that might be pushing it."

"We can get eight," Jack said.

"Okay, lets go eight then,"

The other players, Mitch and Kramer, both bid six. We played the hand, and as we played, Jack and I got the first four books.

"Okay, we might win this after all," I said.

Mitch made a mistake and accidentally cut his partner, which helped me and Jack out in the long run.

"Dammit," Kramer said.

"My bad," Mitch said.

"You probably cost us the game right there," Kramer said.

"Fuck, chill out," Mitch responded.

"We have food on the line, and you want to do some dumb shit like that," Kramer said. Before the game started, me and Jack bet both Kramer and Mitch for canteen. We only bet for three candy bars a piece, but hey food is food. Half the time we were hungry in here too. So this was a pretty big deal in the bigger scheme of things.

I was back in the county for nearly two months after the hospital, and I was waiting for my next court date. My attorney was telling me that I might get probation. I didn't know what to believe at this point.

"Time to lock down, gentlemen," the guard said.

She was on the unit intercom when she called it.

"We still have are game to finish," Mitch said.

"You can finish it later," she said.

She was above us in the control cage. We laid our cards on the table and planned to return to our game tomorrow. I was off to bed, and as I was locking down I had the thought that I wish I wasn't here any more. I felt mentally I was going insane. I will be twenty-two years old this year, I also thought. Man, I wanted out of here so bad, and I wasn't going anywhere fast either. I was stuck right there in that awful place with those awful people. I couldn't believe that this was my life, but I had no choice but to believe it, I thought. I went to lay down, and my mattress had a built in pillow to it. My mattress was blue. I had no sheets for it either. I guess the county thought it would be cheaper to do things this way. My blanket was really no blanket at all. It was a thin white sheet, and it got cold at night. The good thing I guess is the fact that I had a radio. My radio was given to me by the mental health counselor, Sherry. She gives one to all the mental health inmates who are under her care. For Christmas she also gave me a pair of slippers. I still have them, but they are in my property somewhere. I guess if I really wanted them I could write and see if I could get them back, but I had no desire to do so though, so I didn't. Lock down was early. We had to be in our cells by eight o'clock at night. They passed out medications to us at nine o'clock at night. I didn't want the medication I was on because it made me gain so much weight. They had me on depikote still, and I wouldn't be surprised if it was messing up my liver.

"Meds?" the nurse asked.

She was doing her rounds. She had blond hair and green eyes, and she was short and chubby.

"Yes," I said.

I was only med compliant because I wanted probation so badly. I was on depikote, fifteen hundred milligrams of it too. I weighed a little over two hundred and seventy pounds. I was large, that was for certain. I didn't want to be, but I was, and right now there was nothing that I could do about it. So I took my medication, and I called it a night.

The next day we were served breakfast through our hatches, and the guards passed out the food. I had a hard boiled egg and sausage squares. I ate my food and went back to lay down. I put my radio over my ears and listened to some tunes. I waited until the porter came around to pick up my tray. The guards returned to open the hatch for the porter, and I began throwing paper out of my cell. I started throwing crayons, shampoo, and conditioner out of my cell. I began yelling too.

"I want to kill myself! I want to die! Fuck all you guards, you hate me anyways! Fuck you all!"

I kept throwing all my belongings out of my cell. I was angry at everyone.

"Bower, you need to stop that right now," the guard said.

The guard was tall, and young, and he had brown hair.

"Stop that right now, Bower!"

"No!"

"Bower, don't make us come in there," he said.

"What are you going to do about it?"

I had the blanket around my neck, and I began threatening to hang myself.

"You won't save me. No one can save me," I said.

"Don't do it, Bower."

I began choking myself with my blanket that was thin enough to be a sheet.

"Fuck you!"

I was tightening the blanket now. The guard got on his radio and called for back up. In the matter of seconds more guards showed up, and they were all outside my door now. "Be careful, he threw shampoo on the floor, and you don't want to slip," the cage said.

She said it from the intercom, and she was watching everything from the cage. I went to lay on my bed while I was choking myself, and the guard opened my door. I heard the sound of his keys rattling. Not soon after they were prying my hands off of the blanket.

136

"Fuck you," I said.

"Let go, Bower."

"No, fuck you," I said.

"Let go of the blanket, Bower."

The guard finally got the blanket free, and he began to take it away piece by piece. When he did he then pulled out his handcuffs.

"Put your hands behind your back, Bower," he said.

Three other guards were in my cell. I was lying on my bed face first. They grabbed both my arms and put my hands behind my back, and then they placed me in cuffs. From there they escorted me to booking where I would be watched twenty-four seven in a green security smock until I was stable enough to return to my unit.

Chapter 12 Hole Time

I was sent to a sub day cell in the county jail. A sub day cell is a single man cell, and I came out by myself for one hour each day. I showered by myself, and I only had one other person as a neighbor. Other than that, the guards didn't care what I did. As long as I wasn't causing trouble.

"Bower, you want your hour out?"

"Yes," I said.

The guard spoke to me through the silver microphone connected to the wall in my cell. It was silver, and it had a button on it, so I could contact them. The guard popped my cell door, and I came out to sit down in the square. The square was the only space that I had available to move around in. It was an eight foot by ten foot square, shower included. If I wanted to shower, I had to do it during my one hour out. If I wanted to clean my cell, I also had to do that during my hour out. I was not allowed to bring in my cleaning supplies from the sub day area. I had to leave those for the guards to pick up when they wanted them in return. I had a view of the general population from my sub day. I would watch other inmates walk around and play cards or exercise with each other. The days were slow, and there was nothing to do. I guess I had to hurry up and wait. There was a book cart, however, and I would read when I wanted to read.

"Bower, your time is up," the guard said.

I could tell the guard was a female because of her voice.

"Okay, let me put these cleaning supplies back," I said.

"Okay, hurry up, because your neighbor is coming out next," she said.

"Okay," I said.

I was placing the spray bottle on the sub day counter.

"Okay, I am done," I said.

I shut the cell door behind me, and my neighbor was motioned to be let out. I often slept all day because there wasn't much to do. So I would lay down and get some shut eye. I knew one thing about lock up, and that was there was a lot of sleep involved. I hated sleeping all day, because it was depressing. It was sad really—all there was to do was sleep. Especially if you were on your own, and I was on my own. I didn't have anyone to play cards with, and I didn't have anyone to exercise with. No, I had no one, and I knew it too.

"Johnson."

139

I could hear her voice on his intercom through the wall.

"What?"

"You're up," she said.

"Okay."

Johnson sounded old, because he was old. He was an old black man from Mississippi, and he had the accent too. I had three Kit Kat bars in my cell, and a few Kool Aid packets.

"Hey man, how are you doing?"

I was standing at my cell door, and I wanted to make conversation.

"Well, not so good," he said. "I hate it here."

He had his head in his lap.

Johnson was in his sixties, and I think he suffered from Alzheimer's.

"Here you go," I said.

I slid him a Kit Kat bar through the bottom of the door.

"Gee thanks," he said.

"No problem," I said.

"What do I owe ya, boss?"

"A smile," I said.

"I can do that," he said.

Johnson ate the Kit Kat bar with a smile on his face, and it made my day. I enjoyed his smile because I didn't see many people smile in jail. I needed that to feel human again.

"Can I have another one, boss?"

I couldn't say no.

"Sure," I said.

I slid him another Kit Kat bar.

"Here you go," I said.

"Thanks boss."

I never quite understood why he called me boss. I just didn't get it. Maybe it wasn't for me to get. It could have been a generational thing, or maybe it was just a Mississippi thing. Who knew, but I didn't ask him in fear of offending him. I decided that each time I had a candy bar from the canteen, I would save it just for him. I did this as a gesture of thanks, because he smiled for me. I was pleased when I saw him smile. It made me feel like I was worth something. Also Johnson appreciated my kindness, and I could tell he didn't do it to use me. No, I noticed how sincere he was, and that led me to give to him generously.

"Thanks boss," he said.

I did this for four months, and each time it was with

a Kit Kat bar. He loved it, and I enjoyed watching him smile as he ate the chocolate from his fingertips. Not soon after he was gone. I don't know what ever happened to him. He just one day got up and left. I guess his time was up, and he was called to better things. I will never know where he went, but I do know I enjoyed seeing his smile while eating the gift I gave him.

The days were very slow for me, and I often slept during the day. Then I would wake during the night. It was safe to assume I was some kind of vampire or some type of mythical creature. Or maybe just an inmate with a number to my name. I had been in the hole for a while now, and I began to become familiar with the guards. They knew me, and I knew them. At times they were very respectful to me, and I really enjoyed days when they would come to my cell just to talk to me. Not all of them were like that, but a few were. The few that were showed concern for me, and they cared for me. I wasn't sure if they were the same in prison or not. However, I really didn't want to find out. I kept my fingers crossed for me not to go to prison. Soon after I had a next door neighbor. He was white, and he had blond hair and blue eyes. He was much taller than me. He was about six foot three or so.

"What do they call you?"

He was talking to me through the cell door.

"Austin," I said.

"I'm Chris," he said.

"What are you in for?"

"Robbery," I said.

I was standing at my cell door now.

"You?"

"I'm in for reckless driving, and having some meth in my pocket," he said.

"No, shit," I said."Where are you from?"

"I'm from Colorado," Chris said. "You?"

"I'm from California," I said.

"What the fuck brought you out to Lincoln?"

"I would ask you the same question," I said. "No, but I was brought out here by my parents."

"You were young?"

"Ya," I said.

"Well, I'm going to go back to my book," Chris said.

"Okay, talk to you later," I said.

"Ya, talk to you later."

I did the same routine on a daily basis, and I really hated where I was at. You can't really get used to an environment like this. It's just very abnormal, and people aren't the same. I spent an entire year in the hole. The two inmates I did all my time with were Johnson and Chris. I also did my time with some gay guy named Keki. Imagine that, his name was Keki. I didn't talk to him much. After I found out he was gay and he was so open about it, it started to worry me. And I'm not saying all gay people are like this, but he was. Keki began asking me if I liked men, and I didn't like questions like that. I was straight, and will always be straight. So the question caught me by surprise, and from there on I avoided him. He could tell I didn't want to talk, so we didn't.

Chapter 13 Court

In the 1980's observations and studies in many states indicated that an increasing number of discharged mental patients were ending up in jails.

As March 23, 2010 arrived I laid on my mattress, and I continued to ponder what would happen next in my life. Would I go to prison, or would I get probation? I had a lot of questions that were unanswered. Nevertheless my mother continued to tell me to keep my eyes on Christ. It was very difficult to do at times because I had no fellowship. I also had no pastor to visit with. I had been in the sub day section for over a year now. I was lost, and I had no direction to where I was headed in life. I was a high school graduate; however, I was a convicted criminal as well. At least I thought I was, unless I was pardoned or something, and I didn't know about it. Regardless I was here now, and here I would stay until something happened, whether that be shipped upstate or receiving probation. It just wasn't clear to me. I had court three times since my first arrival at the county, one of which I was convicted by all charges. I was still here, and they had me where they wanted me. Who knows, maybe they didn't want me here, but it sure felt like it.

"Bower."

"Ya," I said.

"Get up, you're going to court."

This was my moment of reality, and my moment of truth. I wasn't ready for this, and I didn't feel ready for it either. I was leaning on probation from all the talk that was floating around. I myself was unsure. Only time would tell I guess, and that time was nearing. The guard who came to escort me was tall, and large, and he had brown hair.

"Place your hands through the hatch, Bower," he said.

I did as he instructed, and he opened the door and put the full body chain suit on me.

"When you getting out of here, Bower? You've been here a while."

I looked out the door while he was finishing my leg restraints.

"Ya, I know," I said. "I can't wait to leave either."

He shut the door, and then he began walking as I followed close behind him. The walk was long, and we had to clear a lot of doors just to get to the courtroom. First my door, and then the sub day door. Then we had to go through the general population housing door. From there was a hallway, and from there was another door. Too many doors if you ask me. A lot of clearance was needed too. We couldn't move until zero traffic was in the hallway and until the control tower said it was okay to move. The county building was connected to the county jail, and it seemed to work hand in hand like that. We arrived at the main court door, and the guard had to push a button and pass a security check.

"Kemptner," he said.

He was speaking to control.

"I have one with me to district," he said.

"Okay, you're clear," the box said.

There was also a camera in front of me. The camera was stationed near the door where the county jail was coming into the county building. Once we entered the county building, the guard instructed me to stay quiet. The county building had lawyers and judges all stationed in different offices. Kemptner and I were moving down a long hallway that turned into a row of offices. As we came closer to the courtroom that I would be in, the guard had me wait in a small white room. The room was tagged with graffiti that consisted of gang signs and other gang symbols. I saw crip and blood drawings, along with Mexican graffiti as well. I saw a thirteen carved into the seat that I was seated on. The seat was built in a square, made of a cement block.

"Bower," he said. "Come with me."

I stood up, and I followed him out into the courtroom. This time I already saw the judge seated on his throne. He was there before I had to do the entire 'all rise' thing. I guess that was the privilege you had if you were a judge. You can make people sit or stand whenever you wanted to. I saw my attorney, and I walked over to him and a vacant chair, and I sat down.

"It's looking good," he said. "The judge is granting you probation."

Mac was telling me this while he had his hand over the microphone.

"Mr. Bower," Judge Mass said.

Judge Mass was the district court judge, and I had been working with him ever since Judge Chaos sent my case to district court.

"Yes, your honor," I said.

"It looks like we have found a solution for you," Mass said.

He was speaking with his hands on the desk.

"It looks like the district attorney's office has worked out a deal," he said. "We will be giving you probation. How do you feel about this?"

"Good," I said.

"Very well then," he said. "You will have criteria to follow while you are on probation."

148

"One, you may not consume drugs or alcohol, and you will be drug tested," he said.

"You will be tested for regular testing, twice a week. Two, you will take all medications required to your mental health. Three, you will follow the program guidelines, and undertake drug rehabilitation. Four, you may not be around other felons, and/or drugs or firearms. Five, you will be on probation for three years, by Nebraska state law requirements."

As he finished, I looked to the right of me, and I saw my mother in the courtroom behind the pews.

"Mr. Bower, do you have any questions?"

"No, your honor, I have no questions," I said.

"Mr. Mac?"

"No, your honor," Mac said.

"Mrs. Jerkenson?"

"No, your honor," Jerkenson said.

"Okay then," Mass said.

"Let's schedule the next court hearing, shall we?"

"I have August 9th, 2010," Mass said.

"Your honor," I said.

"Yes, Mr. Bower?"

"That's my birthday."

"Very well then," he said.

"Mrs. Jerkenson, do you have any objection for a later date?"

"No, your honor," Mrs. Jerkenson said.

"Mr. Mac?"

"No, your honor," he said.

"Very well then," he said. "The date scheduled for his probation hearing is going to be August 9th Do I have any objection?"

There was a moment of silence.

"Court dismissed," he said.

Judge Mass looked down on me from his throne.

"Good luck, Mr. Bower," he said.

From there I was escorted back to my cell.

Chapter 14 Probation

In 1955 there was one psychiatric bed for 300 Americans. Since 2005 there is one psychiatric bed for 3,000 Americans.

As I left the county jail, I was larger than when I first went in. I weighed in at two hundred and eighty pounds. I was placed into a program that had very little services. The program was called the Pier program, which stood for *Proactive intense environmental recovery*. It is a program that targets mental health programming in the community. What they failed to realize is I just spent the past year in solitary confinement. I had no sense of direction and no want to do anything really, including probation. Sure probation sounded good for the most part, but I wanted nothing to do with it, let alone the drug testing. The drug testing meant I would have to wake up in the early morning and make a phone call to the probation center, and if I was called in, I would have to find my own way down to the center, whether that meant taking a bus, or finding a ride, or simply walking. I was fat now, and I was still on medications I wasn't supposed to be on. I gained eighty pounds from the medication alone. Nevertheless, it never hurt to try. I was with a Pier worker, and her name was Shelby. We drove in her car all the way to my new apartment from the courthouse. I was surprised to find out they wanted me in my own apartment. I thought I was going to drug rehabilitation, but I guess they changed their minds about it or something. I had my large bag from county property with me. It was a clear, big plastic bag.

"Okay, Austin, this is your place," Shelby said.

She walked me up the steps into my new apartment. My apartment was located on fourteenth and D Street. The neighborhood was bad, and it looked to be drug infested.

Shelby had short cut brown hair and green eyes. She was short and chubby with a fat neck. I thought she was larger than me.

"Okay, so what do I do?"

"Well, we have to file some paperwork, and I will need you to come with me," she said.

"I just want to lay down," I said.

"You don't want to get out?"

"Not really," I said.

"Why not?"

"I just don't. I rather lay down and sleep."

"Well, you just can't lay down and sleep," she said.

"Yes, I can."

"You don't even have a bed yet," she said.

152

"I will lay on the floor."

"No, that's not an option. You need to come with me."

"I don't want to go with you."

"Austin, you don't have a choice, unless you want to go back to the jail," she said.

"No, I don't want to go back there either," I said.

"Well, come on then," she said.

"Can't I just stay?"

"No! Now, let's go," she said.

"No, I'm just going to stay here," I said.

"Okay, you stay here then, and I will do your paperwork without you."

"Okay."

I was laying on the floor, and my property bag from the county jail was laying next to me. It was a large, clear bag, and I had paper and clothing, along with a few canteen items, which included a deck of playing cards, a comb, and some candy I hadn't opened yet. I laid on the floor of my new apartment, and I began to fall asleep. I was tired of everything, and that included being told what to do. My apartment was small, and it had one bathroom and one bedroom. I guess the good thing about it was the dishwasher because that meant I didn't have to do any dishes. The machine would do it all for me.

I began to explore my new life while being on probation with pain, rather than hope. I still felt very confined, and who wouldn't? I just came out of lock up. I was locked up for nearly eighteen months, and I was told what to do all of the time. Now I had some freedom, and I was still being told what to do. That was more of a challenge in my mind. When they said probation, I must not of fully understood what they meant. I didn't know it would mean going to groups and taking drug testing. I mean I did, but I didn't at the same time. About an hour passed by, and Shelby soon returned.

"Austin," Shelby said. "It's me, Austin."

She was at my door calling my name.

"Austin, can I come in?"

I got up to let her in.

"Okay, I got all of your paperwork done," she said. "No thanks to you. You will need to call the probation center tomorrow because you need to see if you're selected for testing."

"I have to call every day?"

"Yes," she said. "Every day. Your probation officer is coming to see you shortly."

"Okay," I said.

She had an odd look on her face.

"I would clean up if I were you," she said.

"Why?"

"Because your property is all over the floor," she said.

"I have nowhere to put it."

"Put it in your closet."

"I don't care about that," I said.

"Well, you should."

She stood on her tip toes when she said it.

"Well, I don't," I said.

"Okay, I'm not going to argue with you about it. I have to go. I will be by tomorrow."

She was leaning on the door now and preparing to leave.

"Okay, bye Austin."

She was headed out the door, and then she turned around quickly.

"Oh Austin, your probation officer will be here in thirty minutes," she said.

"So stay awake."

"Okay," I said.

I went back to the floor to lay down, and I did nothing. All that I did was lay there. I didn't care about a thing. All I wanted to do was sleep, and it was all that I did in the county. So I sort of just got used to it. The time went by, and I could hear someone at my door.

"Knock! Knock! knock!" the door rang out.

"Who is it?"

"It's Casey, your probation officer," she said. "Can I come in?"

"Sure," I said.

I let her into my apartment. She had blond hair and blue eyes. She was tall and had a strong build. She was wearing a yellow shirt and blue jeans.

"You, must be Austin," she said.

"Yes, I am Austin."

"Okay, well Austin I need to check your apartment for any drugs or firearms," she said.

"Be my guest," I said.

So I let Casey into the kitchen, and she looked inside my refrigerator for any alcohol.

"Great, no alcohol."

Then she looked into the cabinets.

"Very good, they are empty," she said.

She began to move towards the living room, which was empty as well. After the living room, she moved towards my bedroom, which had no bed in the room.

"Let me look into your closet," she said.

156

She slid the closet door open.

"Okay, great, nothing in here," she said. "Let me look into your bathroom."

She walked over to the bathroom, and she moved the shower curtain. Then she opened the medicine cabinet, and that was empty as well.

"Great, everything looks good, Austin. What's up with all the stuff on your floor?"

"Those are my belongings, from the county," I said.

"Okay, well make sure you pick them up," she said.

"Okay," I said.

"Here is my card, Austin."

"Just so you know, your code is hungry hippo three," she said. "So if you hear that code, be sure you come down to the probation office to drug test."

"Okay."

"You will be called twice a week," she said. "Any questions?"

"What time do I call at?"

"Six in the morning. Any more questions?"

"No," I said.

"Okay, great Austin, I will see you next week," she said.

After Casey left, I went back to lay down and go to

sleep. I slept all the way until the evening, and as I was sleeping I heard a knock at my door.

"Hi Austin, I have your medication here for you," she said.

I opened the door to see who it was.

"Hi, I am Molly," she said.

She had a smile on her face.

"You guys bring me my medication?"

"Yes, we do, Austin," Molly said.

She was tall with brown hair and brown eyes. She was wearing a Batman t-shirt.

"So how are you feeling?"

"Okay, I guess," I said. "I'm tired."

"Okay, take these pills," she said.

She was watching me as I was taking my medication.

I had a cup of water in my right hand.

"Okay," I said.

"Okay, Austin, I will see you later," she said.

I shut the door to my apartment, and I laid back down. I had no food to eat, and I went hungry the first night that I was out, and I had no money either. With no money, I couldn't buy anything. So I stuck it out hoping that eventually something would come my way. I slept the entire night, and did so on my living room floor. The very next day, a knock was at my door. I went to answer it, and I was tired. I started rubbing my eyes, and I opened the door.

"Hey, Austin, how are you?"

It was Shelby again.

"I have your meds here for you," she said.

Shelby had my medication in a small bag.

I grabbed a cup of water, and she handed me my medication. I took my water, and I took my medication, and I swallowed my pills.

"So, did you call your probation office?"

"No," I said.

"Well, why not?"

"Because I don't have a phone," I said.

"Okay... well we better get you one then," she said. "Can you talk to your payee about giving you money for a phone?"

"Yes," I said.

"Okay, make sure that you do," she said. "You don't want to go back to the county jail."

"I know."

I was getting tired of everyone throwing the county jail in my face. My day went by slowly because all I did was remain in my apartment. My apartment was dark, because I had all the lights off. Eventually I decided to get out of my apartment and walk up to the gas station. I had no money, but I figured if I asked someone for a few dollars, I would receive a few dollars. The gas station was only three blocks away from where I lived. As I was walking, I recognized someone. It was my homeboy Jack, and he was standing outside of a house smoking a cigarette.

"Jack," I said. "Hey Jack."

I got his attention, and I was walking alongside a tree and a garbage can. I was in view of a mailbox in front of me. The apartments were in a row, and the houses looked worn down.

"Austin? Is that you?"

He paused for a second.

"Holy shit," he said. "They really gave you probation?"

"Yes sir," I said.

"So what are you doing?"

"Nothing."

"Do you want a drink?"

"I better not," I said. "I'm on probation."

"Come on, just one drink?"

"Okay sure," I said. "I will have one drink. What do

you got?"

"I have rum or I have Jim Beam," he said.

"Jim Beam sounds good," I said.

"Okay, come with me," he said.

I followed him into the house.

"So who's house is this?"

"Mine," he said.

"Really?"

"What, you don't believe me?"

"It's not that," I said.

"No, it's my girlfriend's," he said. "I was only fucking with you."

He had a cigarette in his mouth while laughing, and his mouth was muffled while he was talking from the cigarette. Jack had a pony tail, and a new tattoo on his neck. The tattoo on his neck read '*fifty one fifty.*'

"You like my new tattoo?"

"Ya, it's cool," I said.

"It stands for the crazy code out in California," he said. "You know that I'm from San Francisco, don't you?"

"Ya, you told me," I said.

"Cool," he said.

161

He was grabbing the bottle of Jim Beam. The bottle was large and made of glass.

"Isn't it a little early to be drinking?"

"No, drink up," he said.

He poured the whiskey in a cup.

"Here you go," he said.

I began to drink, and I drank the entire cup in under two minutes.

"How are you feeling?"

"Good," I said.

"Do you want a tattoo?"

"Sure," I said.

"My brother is asleep in his room," he said. "Once he comes out, I will ask him to tat you up."

"Okay," I said.

I sat there on the sofa drunk, and I was still drinking. His brother woke up about an hour later.

"Hey Frank," Jack said.

"Ya," Frank said.

They were talking from other rooms. I was in the living room with Jack, while Frank was in his bed room. We could hear him moving around in the other room.

"Austin wants a tattoo," he said.

"Does he have money?"

"Do you have money?"

"Yes," I said.

"Yes!"

"Okay, how much does he have?"

"I don't know," Jack said.

"How much do you have, Austin?"

Jack was speaking to me while sipping on his rum.

"I need to go to my payee," I said.

"He will get the money from his payee," Jack said.

"That's good enough for me," Frank said. "Let's do it."

Frank came out of his room with a tattoo gun and some bottles of ink. Frank had on a blue shirt and a black baseball cap.

"Okay, you ready?"

"Ya," I said.

"What do you want?"

"I don't know," I said.

"What's your name?"

"Austin Bower," I said.

163

"Okay, let's do an A and a B on your neck," he said. "Then I want to do one on your arm. Do you want one on your arm?"

"Ya, my sister's name," I said.

"Okay, what's her name?"

"Drucella," I said.

"Okay, we will do her name," he said.

"You will have to lay on your back for the tattoos on your neck," he said.

"Okay."

I got on my back, and Frank began to tattoo my neck. Frank used a needle from his gun, and I didn't know if it was clean or not.

"Is the needle clean?"

"Ya, it's clean," he said.

"Okay."

Frank began to do all three of my tattoos, and the neck hurt more than the arm did. He took his time with the ink and the gun, and he would dip the ink into the needle. The gun looked to be homemade. It looked like it was made of parts from a CD player. He moved from my neck to my arm, and then he finished from there. It took about an entire hour for him to finish.

"Okay, all set," he said.

164

I was drunk still as I was laying on the floor. Frank was getting up off of the floor.

"That will cost you fifty dollars, once you get your money," Frank said.

"How about one more tattoo?"

Frank paused for a second.

"Of what?"

"Something," I said.

"Okay, where at?"

"On my hand," I said.

"I know what you can do," Jack said.

Jack was seated on the sofa.

"A skull with a bandanna on it."

"Okay," Frank said. "Take a seat in this chair."

I sat down on an old metal chair. The chair had rust all over it, and the seat was yellow. Frank began to give me the tattoo on my hand. Frank was on the floor seated in front of me, and he was doing the same routine that he did before. He would dip the needle and wipe at the ink. He had with him a white wash cloth, and he would run lines and make strong edges.

"Okay, it's looking good," he said. "I am almost done."

He continued to apply the ink to my skin. My neck was still hurting a little from the tattoo Frank just gave me.

"Okay," he said. "I'm all done."

"Okay," I said.

I looked at my hand, and it was swollen, but the tattoo looked good.

"What time is it?"

Jack looked at his phone.

"It's noon," Jack said.

"I better get going," I said.

I was still drunk, and I was headed back to my apartment. I couldn't remember why I wanted to go to the gas station. I was walking alongside my apartment parking lot.

"Austin," Casey said.

I was screwed, I thought, because I could taste the alcohol on my breath, which meant she would be able to smell the alcohol.

"Yes," I said.

She approached me. She had on a red shirt and black pants.

"Austin, where were you this morning? You were called in," she said.

166

"I don't have a phone," I said.

"Your breath smells like alcohol," she said. "Have you been drinking? Is that why you didn't show up? Austin, I need to call the police. You need to come with me," she said.

I followed her to her car, and she stood outside her vehicle. She was talking on her phone. Her car was parked in the back parking lot behind a tree.

"The police are on their way," she said. "Austin, you messed up, bud. Not even a full week. You messed up."

The police eventually showed up and cuffed me. The officer had a blue uniform on and black running shoes. He was wearing sunglasses that were red and black. The officer had the door open to the back seat. Casey was standing in front of me bent over, while I was seated in the back seat of the cruiser.

"Maybe in jail you can think about what you did," she said.

She shut the door, and after that the police sent me back to corrections.

Chapter 15 Back at County

Those with mental health diagnosis in recent studies show that they die 25 years before the rest of the general population. One out of ten reasons for why this happens is due to incarceration.

I was back in the county jail, and at this point the guards were familiar with who I was. They treated me a little differently than when I first arrived. One, they knew I had a mental health condition, and some of them even knew I was autistic.

"Bower, what are you doing back, bud?"

The guard's name was Maddox. He was six foot two, and he had a strong build. He kept his head shaved clean.

"I don't know," I said.

"Well, you're here now, so let's try to make the best of it," he said.

The officer that brought me in placed his red and black sunglasses behind his ears.

"He is here on a probation violation," he said.

"Okay, we got it," Maddox said.

I was standing at the counter.

"Let's get you stripped out, Austin," Maddox said.

"Okay."

I followed his lead to the strip out room, and I felt that Maddox favored me a little. I knew him for eighteen months. We both had a good report with one another. I remember one time he gave me an extra piece of pizza off of a tray that wasn't being used. Maddox stripped me out, and he sent me to the holding cell. From there I watched as first shift was starting to leave and second shift was taking over.

"Okay, Bower, I'm out of here," Maddox said. "You take care."

"You too," I said.

I thought Maddox was cool for a cop. He didn't go out of his way to target anybody like some of the guards did. No, he was different, and he displayed that he was different. Second shift began to settle in, and from there they began preparing my move to the special needs unit.

"Bower, your escort is here," he said.

"Okay."

The guard was tall and large with blond hair. He looked to be in his thirties.

"You ready, Bower?"

"Yes," I said.

"Okay, let's get this show on the road," he said.

He had a giddy way to his personality. He seemed to be happy for some reason, and I wasn't sure why, but he was. He opened the door and led me down the hall. We both passed by three doors on the way to the special needs unit. He opened the unit door and led me inside.

"You're on the bottom tier, Bower," he said. "You're in cell four."

He pointed at the cell, and the control tower popped my door. I went in, and I locked down in my room. No one was out of their cells, and everyone was locked down. I laid on my mattress, and I started thinking how this sucked. I couldn't believe I was back in the county. I wasn't even out for an entire week. One thing I realized, though, is I could go back to sleep whenever I wanted, and that is exactly what I did.

Chapter 16 Sentencing

There are 2.3 million people currently incarcerated in the united states. There are 1,719 state prisons, 102 federal prisons, 942 juveniel correctional facilities, and 3,283 local jails. Along with 79 immigration detention facilities, Military prisons, and civil commitment centers.

March 8th, 2011 the courtroom was furnished with beautiful oak wood and green padding. The chairs were oak and had green padding too. I was seated in front of the judge, and my attorney was seated next to me. The district attorney was at her seat. My mother sat in the front row of the courtroom, and my probation officer sat next to my mother. My mother was wearing a nice outfit that had butterflies for the theme. Casey was wearing black pants and a white long sleeve shirt. The judge had our attention, and he began to speak.

"Okay, this is the matter of State of Nebraska verses Austin Bower," Mass said. "CRO9-1128. And you are Mr. Bower, right?"

"Yes, sir," I said.

He had no smile on his face.

"Okay, Mr. Bower," he said. "The record reflects that on February 11, 2011 you appeared before me."

I was looking down at my hands playing with my

thumbs.

"At that time you admitted to me that you violated certain terms of your intensive supervision probation," he said.

I looked up at the judge.

"I have an updated presentence investigation report, and I am now ready to proceed with sentencing," Mass said.

Jerkenson was looking at her file that she had in front of her.

"I received a letter from your mother," he said. "And I received a letter from an Ashely Phinox, which I read them both. Both letters were added to the presentencing report. Before we got started here today, Ms. Jerkenson, Ms. Casey, and Mr. Mac were in my office," he said.

"Mr. Mac reported to me that the other option, CenterPoint, was unavailable," Mass said. "They reported to Mr. Mac that they had no space for you and that you wouldn't fit their program Am I right, Mr. Mac?"

"I believe so," Mac said.

"Okay, the question is should the probation of March 23, 2010 as amended August 9, 2010, should that probation be revoked? Any comments, Ms. Jerkenson?"

172

"Your Honor, I am asking that it be revoked," she said.

"Any comments Mr. Mac?"

"Your Honor, I am asking that the probation should not be revoked," Mac said.

"Okay, Mr. Bower, I am going to do two things here," Mass said.

"Number one, I am going to decide if I should revoke your probation order. If I revoke the probation order, that doesn't mean you won't get probation and it doesn't mean you will get probation. It just means I will sentence you, just like I could have sentenced you back on March 23, 2010. Do you understand?"

"Uh-huh," I said.

"Okay," Mass said.

"I find on the information before me that the ISP order of March 23, 2010 as modified August 9, 2010 should be, and here by is revoked. Ms. Jerkenson, are you aware of any corrections or updates to this presentence investigation?"

"No, your Honor," Jerkenson said.

"Mr. Mac, are you aware of any changes or corrections?"

"No, your Honor," Mac said.

"Okay, any comments for sentencing, Ms.

173

Jerkenson?"

"No, your Honor," Jerkenson said.

"Mr. Mac?"

"Thank You," Mac said. "On Austin's behalf, I think we told the court our options are pretty well running out," he said.

"And I don't have anything else to suggest, but I think a long term dual diagnosis program that would keep him isolated from his peers that have gotten him into trouble in the past. We knew that CenterPoint was a good program that would provide these services. They have now indicated they do not think Austin would be a good fit for their program. We don't have any other facility or program to offer the court," Mac said.

"Thank you," Mass said.

"Mr. Bower, do you have any comments to make in respect to what I should do?"

"Your Honor," I said, "I am really sorry you had to see me here again. And I'm just really sorry I let you down."

Mass looked down at me, and he began to speak.

"Are you ready for me to tell you what I'm going to do?"

"Yes," I said.

"Number one," Mass said, "I don't want you to feel

174

you let me down," he said. "You may of let your family down. To me, more importantly, you've let yourself down. You have to realize you have to do these things for you, not for your mom, not for Judge Mass, but for you," he said.

"Yeah," I said.

"The order I received from Ms. Casey, your probation officer stated that other people came into your apartment and took advantage of you," he said.

"Yeah," I said.

"You know, and I know, and every one in here knows that you have special needs. That doesn't mean you can't be successful, in my opinion."

"I know," I said.

"But you have to do it for yourself," he said.

"Okay."

"The letter Mr. Mac sent me, dated yesterday," Mass said.

"He met with a lot of people, and one of the lines says after they reviewed all these things, everything they reviewed suggests a possibility that no reasonable options are left for you. I don't agree with that. I know there are options out there. However, the options I have are limited, and I've used all my options with you. So I don't believe probation is appropriate at this time," he said.

"I know, I know," I said.

"Your position is that Mr. Hawkboy beat him up, and you didn't beat any one up, and you were just there. But I know you were part of that also. You know and I know you have special needs. I also know you were under the influence of drugs, and that doesn't make it right. But being under the influence and your special needs makes you more usable, if you will, by somebody else. That, however, doesn't change the crime. I sentenced Mr. Hawkboy to something like 12 to 15 years. I believed he was the primary moving force of the crime. The court finds it is necessary for Mr. Bower to be imprisoned for the protection of the public. You still do things illegal. You haven't beaten anyone up, but you use drugs. I don't believe you would be able to adhere to the terms of probation, and a lesser sentence would depreciate the seriousness of your crime or promote disrespect to the law. It is there for the judgment and sentence that Austin E. Bower be committed to an institution under jurisdiction of the department of correctional services for the period of no less than five years, nor more than eight years, no part of which shall be in solitary confinement, except for violation of prison rules. You shall pay the cost of this action. You must serve two and one half years minus credit for time served for parole. And you must serve four years minus credit for timed served for mandatory discharge. You will have DNA testing done, which will be at the cost of you. You have thirty days to file

176

a direct appeal, Anything else, Mr. Mac?"

"I have nothing else," Mac said.

"Ms. Jerkenson?"

"No, your Honor," she said.

"You can go back with him if you'd like, Mr. Mac," Mass said. "Or you can talk to him later."

"I can talk to him later," Mac said.

"What's that mean? I don't get it," I said. "Am I going to prison?"

"You are," Mass said.

I was escorted by the bailiff and walked back through the large wooden door. I watched as the Judge remained seated at his throne. I began to think that things would only get worse from here. I guess only time would tell.

Chapter 17 Prison

An estimated 56 percent of state prisons, 45 percent of federal prisons, and 64 percent of local jails with in the united states is the percentage of inmates diagnosed with one or more mental health problems in the United States.

I was transferred to the Lincoln Correctional Center, through county jail transport, and the two officers were Jefferson and Done. The facility looked large, and it looked like a military base. The guards had me riding in the back of the vehicle while both guards rode up front. Two officers occupied the vehicle. One drove and the other rode passenger. They were both having conversations with one another quietly. I had no idea what it was about; it was too quiet for me to hear what they were saying. Plus, a piece of plastic glass blocked them from me, for various reasons of course, such as spitting or head butting. We drove about four miles, from facility to facility. Upon arrival a large gated metal door lifted up after the driving officer went to a small security box to contact the staff inside.

There were cameras on the vehicle of the mini-van, and it was a mini-van that was recreated into a jail van. I was arriving to my final destination, otherwise known as prison. So the gate opens, and the van enters, and on the inside were rails and steps and there was a wheelchair ramp too. The driveway to the inside entrance was large and wide, but not too long. The county officer slowly drove in the van.

"Okay, Bower, this is your stop," Jefferson said.

"Okay," I said.

I never thought I would be entering prison. I was afraid, scared, and worried. My first thought was Hawkboy would attempt to take me out—you know, kill me. I thought the worst that would happen, would be getting stabbed or jumped. I wasn't ready for a fight, and the medications I was on made me weigh over three hundred pounds. Believe it, I was fat. I was a straight fat ass, and I hated being fat too. I just hated it. The thought of it was up setting. The worst part about it was it wasn't from eating. It was from the medications. I was escorted into a large office by both county officers.

"Name?"

 I was looking around. I was next to six other inmates.

"Name?"

I continued to look around, and I was overwhelmed. The desk was long and wide, and the desk had one computer.

"Hey you, what is your fucking name?"

I became startled.

The women was fat and large with blond hair. She was tall too, probably six foot. Her name tag read, "*Pock*."

I looked at her again.

"My name is Bower," I said.

"Bower, come this way," she said.

I followed the large women, and I went to the other side of the desk.

"I have a series of questions that I need to ask of you," Pock said. "Do you have any mental health history?"

"Yes," I said.

"Okay, what?"

"I have Tourette's syndrome, and I have Bi-Polar," I said. "I also have autism."

"Okay, any thoughts of suicide right now?"

"No," I said.

"Okay, are these your items?"

As my belongings laid on the long desk, there were papers and a shirt along with a pair of shoes and a belt. There was also a book and a few pairs of socks.

"We don't keep things like this here, so you can mail them home or you can trash them. If you mail them home, you will be charged an eight dollar fee, including tax. If you trash them, it's free," Pock said.

"You can trash them, if you want," I said.

She looked at me.

"Well, that's up to you," she said.

I looked at her again.

"Ya, you can trash them," I said

"Okay."

I looked puzzled.

"No wait, you can mail them home."

She looked upset now.

"Which one will it be?"

"You can mail them home."

"Okay, and then that's it, final decision, no turning back?"

"Ya," I said.

"Okay, sign this form here."

I signed the form, and she directed me into another station which was held by a male correctional officer.

"Name?"

"Bower," I said.

This time the guard didn't have to repeat himself, like Pock did.

181

"Okay, take off all of your clothing, and put this blue shampoo in your hair," he said. "Make sure you wash for five minutes. Before we do that, though, I need to search you."

The guard did not hesitate at all, not even a flinch.

"Take off your clothes," he said.

I began taking my clothing off with the feeling of humiliation. I was all the way

undressed from my shirt to my underwear.

"Okay, lift up the bottom of your feet," he said.

I did as he asked of me.

"Okay, turn around and spread your cheeks," he said.

I looked puzzled.

"What?"

"It's no different from county jail, you know the drill," he said.

"Okay."

I turned around.

"Bend over," he said.

I looked embarrassed now, and I hesitated.

"I said bend over, God dammit! Now cough!"

I coughed.

"Okay, take your fucking shower, and afterwords you

need to piss in this cup," he said. So I did as instructed with the blue shampoo. I hurried my shower, and then I got dressed. I felt overwhelmed by the entire process. The towel that I used was dry like sandpaper. I put my clothing on, and then I waited for further instruction; The blue suit took his time.

"Okay, you can come in, Bower," he said. "Okay, stand on the scale."

I looked around, and then I stood on the scale.

The scale was making digital noises. The numbers would go back and forth, and then they would slow down to a certain degree.

"Three hundred and three pounds. Wow Bower, you are a fat ass," he said.

He began to laugh and smile at me.

"Okay, stand under the height measure, next to you there, and face forward," he said.

The guard had brown hair and a long nose. He was rather tall too.

I did as he asked.

"Okay, we have you at six foot even," he said.

"Do you have any tattoos?

This time the guard hesitated.

"Hey, just take your shirt off," he said. "Okay, well

let's see what we have here, '*California*' on your back, and we have '*Bower*' on your upper left arm. We also have a '*skull tattoo*' on your left hand. And we have a tattoo of an *A* and a *B* on your neck," he said.

The guard took a very close look at all of my tattoos.

"Okay, we will need to take photos of all of your tattoos. Come over here and face the camera," he said.

The guard took one photo at a time, all the way to the last tattoo.

The guard was coming to a finish.

"Okay Bower, you're all set. Your number is on your card here, *73223,*" he said. "It will be your number for your duration of your sentence."

I looked at my new yellow identification card with my photo on it.

Underneath the photo was my number.

"Okay, next we will have you wait for the case manager to meet with you," he said.

I looked around and I saw an older looking man in a button up shirt and blue jeans sitting at a computer table. At his desk, he had a name tag that said *Elks*. I went over to the small square room where four other inmates were sitting. The room was filthy with the smell of mold. The square room had a bench in it to sit down on. However, a few inmates preferred to stand, rather than to sit. I didn't blame them—anything could happen. Someone could have a knife or a homemade shank.

"Bower," Elks said.

"Yes."

"Come this way. I need to talk to you," he said.

I walked over to the desk, stationed toward the hallway. I slowly walked over to the computer table that held an empty seat, next to the elderly man.

"Okay," he said. "Are there any no contacts on your keep separate list?"

I looked concerned on telling him while other inmates were nearby.

"Yes," I whispered.

"Okay, who?"

"Kevin Hawkboy," I said.

"Okay, I know Hawkboy," he said. "We go way back. I will have him placed on your no contact list."

"Okay," I said.

"Is that it?"

"Ya, that's it."

"Okay, are you in any gang affiliations?"

"No," I said.

Mentally I felt as if I were going crazy; physically there was really nothing that I could do about it. As dreadful as my situation was, what choice did I really have? I mean, I was already here. The case manager was finished and waved his hand over to the guard.

"Okay, let's go," Pock said.

The correctional staff had me wait in a small waiting room. I waited until my transfer. About thirty minutes went by before any real leg action happened. When it did, my real journey would begin. I wasn't ready, and I was unprepared. A blue suit entered the admissions unit, and on his name tag it read Lemon. He was tall and very skinny.

"Okay, you all come with me," Lemon said.

We were currently in the diagnostic and evaluation center, otherwise known as D&E. I was led down a long hallway, I walked the hall and noticed it was very narrow and old; and the hall had mold on the ceiling. There were a lot of pipes running through the walls and ceiling of the hallway as well. The hallway was about a football field in length. When I arrived, I noticed two power doors that were heavy metal, one of which had a microphone established inside the wall next to the key hole. Also a small strip out station was set up for inmates coming and going. I stripped and did the entire embarrassing thing all over again. There was a small white curtain connected to a metal rod. Afterwords I was headed to my unit, and I went through both heavy metal doors. After going through the two large doors, there was a long broad hallway. The hallway had several units connected to it. On my arrival I was sent to unit one, and I noticed about twenty-eight inmates having yard outside. Then I noticed another thirty or so confined in their cells. The units were divided into two units, and on this particular unit I peered outside and noticed pull up bars along with a basketball court and inmates playing basketball. I had no idea what I was going to do. I was uneducated with so many things, gang politics, the rules of the guards, and so many other things. I was a target for certain, and I was also unprepared.

"Fresh Meat!"

"Fresh Meat!"

"Fresh Meat!"

Inmates started yelling.

It was their way to test an inmate to see if they would break or bend, a new inmate in particular. That's just what they did, and it's how they did it.

"Bower," Colmbs said.

"Bower!"

I heard my name, but had no idea who was saying it.

"Bower!"

I continued to hear it, but I had no idea who it was. I

couldn't see him. He must have been in my blind spot or something.

"Bower!"

"God dammit Bower, you don't hear me calling your name?"

I looked behind me, and then I turned around. I noticed the blue suit named Colmbs was calling my name.

"Bower, get your ass over here. We need to take your weight," he said.

I stared for a moment and then replied.

"I already did my weight," I said.

"Well, come do it again," Colmbs said.

He seemed pissed off too.

I walked over to do my weight, and I stepped on the scale across the hall in a small entrance of where the nurse was located. The scale was a portable scale. The nurse was nurse Kelly, and she had red hair and wore glasses.

"Take your boots off," Kelly said.

"Why?"

The guard got snappy with me real quick.

"Take your fucking boots off now, Bower!"

I got off the scale, and I then sat on the floor and

began untying my boots.

"Jesus Bower, do you really need the floor?"

Once I had them off, I stood on the scale.

The scale read '*three hundred, and three.*'

I honest to God had no idea why they wanted me to stand on the scale again. It just made no sense to me. Taking the boots off was the easy part, but putting them back on was the hard part.

"Bower, get the fuck out of my sight, you fucking lard ass!"

I began to walk back to my unit through the small corridor, and I had my head held down. Then things went from bad to worse.

"Bower, you are in cell upper twenty-nine," Colmbs said.

I walked over to lower twenty-five near the stairs and began climbing the steps.

"Bower, upper twenty-nine, can't you hear? Not upper thirty-two, but upper twenty-nine!" Colmbs said, snapping yet again.

"Okay," I said.

"No, it's not okay. You went the wrong way," Colmbs said.

I turned around and began walking toward twenty-nine. When I arrived a big white guy was already bunked in his cell.

"Pop twenty-nine!" Colmbs yelled out.

I tried to open the door by pulling on it, and I couldn't get it open.

"Damn, Bower, what's the hold up?"

"I can't get it open," I said.

"Well try it again! Pop twenty-nine!" Colmbs yelled.

The door popped again making a noise, and this time I twisted the knob to open the door.

"I got the door open," I said.

"Ya, I can see that jack ass. Now lock down," Colmbs said.

I walked in, and I shut the door behind me.

When I walked in I saw three double bunk beds, which only held one person so far. I was the second man in. I also saw a toilet with a metal sink and a funny looking mirror. Inside sat a large white man, and he had a beard that went down to his chest. He had a crew cut haircut, and he had many tattoos on his arms and legs which were visible to me. I didn't say anything at all. I waited for him to break the ice. He was quiet for a while, and time slipped away. It had been over an hour before anyone began a conversation, and I just sat on my bunk.

"So, new guy, what are you in for?" the bearded man asked me with a slight whisper.

190

"Robbery," I said.

"No shit," he said.

"Ya, it was a hard thing to accept too," I said. "That I was coming here."

He looked away.

"And you?"

"And me what?"

"What are you in for?"

"Manslaughter," he whispered.

"Really, who did you kill?"

He looked deep into my presence, especially after I asked that question.

"My wife, on accident," he said.

I was blown away by his words, and a little afraid of him too. I just didn't know how to accept what he just said. I mean, I was supposed to share a cell with this guy. And here he is a killer nonetheless. I was afraid after he told me what he was in for. Who wouldn't be? I felt like I needed to get away from him as soon as possible. But I couldn't let him know that I wanted to get away from him. I would be labeled as a rat if I said I was afraid. So I pondered what I would do; I had a plan to tell the guard that I wanted a room change or something. Later that night chow was called, and I walked up to the guard after I ate my meal, and I ate alone. I tried to avoid other inmates in the meantime.

"Hey sir, can I please move cells or something?"

He looked me up and down. The guard was new to the shift. He wasn't the same one as before.

This blue suit was taller and skinnier than the one prier. The guard's name tag read Peterson. I was whispering in fear I would be overheard by the other inmates.

Peterson had no tolerance and probably thought I was trying to pull a stunt. However, I wasn't. I wanted to be moved badly. I feared for my life.

"Go back to your cell, like the others," he said.

So I headed back to my cell, and no one knew what I asked, thankfully. I tried to make the best of it. I thought to myself, this guy has nothing to lose. Him killing me in my sleep would mean nothing to him at all, I thought. So I went back to my cell for lockdown. I made superficial talk with my cellmate. I didn't really want to know his name, but he told me anyway.

"My name is Max," he said.

I told him my name, and then I moved on to do other things. He received the impression that I didn't want to talk. Which was true because I wanted nothing to do with him. In all fairness, I wanted nothing to do with all of them.

It was my first night, and lights were out. Time started to fly, and it was eleven o'clock at night. I had chest pains that bothered me. I thought I was dying, so I went to my cell door. I began to yell outside of the door. My chest was hurting badly, and it was probably from anxiety—that's all I could think it was from. I wasn't sure, but I needed to know. No response was given by the third shift crew.

"C.O!" I yelled over and over again.

Max was trying to sleep, and the last thing that I wanted to do was anger him.

"Austin," Max said.

He began to instruct me on what to do.

"Pound on that motherfucker, man. That's the only way to get their attention," Max said.

So I began pounding on the door repetitively.

"Bang! Bomb! Bang!"

Over and over again, and eventually a blue suit came out, through the heavy metal door. He looked from a distance at who was making the noise.

"Who's banging?"

"I am sir; I need medical attention please!"

"Why? You sound fine to me," he said.

The blue suit was black with a short haircut, and he was skinny too.

The blue suit walked up the steps; I could hear his boots squeak against the tile.

"What's the problem?"

We were face to face now.

"I need medical attention, sir," I said.

He peered at me momentarily.

"Go to bed or I will write you up for disturbing the peace of others," he said.

"Okay."

As I watched him walk away, I tried to remain calm through it all. So back to bed I went still fearing for my life. I did my best to not let Max know that though. I figured the less Max knew the better. So I went to lie down, and believe me I wanted nothing more than to escape. I noticed Max was breathing and still awake underneath his covers. I felt like having minimum talk or none at all. I was disturbed to know that Max had killed his own wife. I was bothered by the fact, and I did think maybe he is lying to me, just to remain safe himself. Like what if he were to really be a sex offender or something sick like that? That I did not know, all that I had was his word, and right now he was a killer. And I am his next victim; I am his next prey. That is all I could think about, and I couldn't shake the thought of it at all.

Did he have a shank?

194

Did he have a lock in a sock, planning to beat my face in during my sleep?

The not knowing was killing me; it had me under distress. I was confined with this loonie! This loonie!

Jesus, he plans to kill me!

What am I to do??

Okay Austin, calm down. You will be all right. My thoughts were running wild at this point. I need to get out of here, and I need to get out of here now!

"So..." I said. "Just you and me in here."

He was silent for a moment.

"Yep...," he said. "Is that a problem?"

"No..no..no problem. I just.... well, I am just having a hard-"

"Enough!" Max yelled out. "Save it."

I fell silent.

"What, you don't think I know? You going to the guard at chow! You attempting to get the guard's attention?"

He looked me dead in the face, with his head slightly uncovered.

"I know, and you didn't know that I knew, but I did," he said.

I looked at him for a brief moment.

195

"Know what?"

"The fact that you are afraid of me, God dammit! I fucking know!"

Max sounded crazy; his name fit that film perfectly, Mad Max.

Max stood up and hovered over me.

"Get your ass up right now," he said. "Get up, I said!"

He was angry, mad, enraged, and pissed. I think he was past frustrated at this point.

"Get your fucking ass up, right fucking now!"

I just laid there confused and anxious, and I had no idea what he wanted to prove.

"So, you won't get up," he said. "Okay, you plan to pack your shit tomorrow. If you don't pack it, I will pack it for you. Do you understand me?"

I looked at him, and I could tell that he wasn't playing around.

"Okay," I said.

"Tomorrow you will pack your belongings, you got that?" Max said.

"You bet, sir," I said.

Max looked me over for a few moments.

"You don't belong here," Max said.

"What kind of judge would send someone like you here? Do you even know how to fight?"

"No sir," I said.

"Are you mentally ill?"

"I think so," I said.

"With what?"

"I have autism," I said.

"No, I have a stepson with autism. You don't seem autistic to me. They sent you here? Did they know you were autistic?"

"Yes," I said.

"Did you do it?"

"Do what?"

"The robbery, did you do it?"

"No, it was someone else that did it," I said. "I was just there."

"Wow, who was your judge?"

"I rather not talk about this," I said.

"Fair enough. You know, I had a Mexican friend who gave me a bag of dope once. Meth, you ever do that before?"

"Yes," I said.

"Well, anyways, I told him thank you for the dope,

my friend," Max said.

"Ya," I said.

"Well, he said to me, 'I am not your friend, Max. If I were your friend, I would not give you this dope."

Max looked at me and continued.

"You see, Austin, if you think the people here are here to be your friend, think again bud," he said.

I looked at Max with the shadow of the bunks peering over us. The light to the cell was still off. The cell was more relaxed now, and as the night continued I dozed off to sleep. By midnight Max and I were both silent and dead a sleep.

The next morning breakfast was called, and you could see the television in the day hall. The channel to the television was on ESPN. It was showing some highlights of last year's college football championship games. I was waiting in line for the meal server to serve me my breakfast. The inmate porters did the food serving. I was given cereal and toast with a cup of 2% milk. I went to sit down to eat my breakfast, and a few other guys came to sit down next to me.

"So, what are you in for?"

He was slender and short, and he didn't seem to have a strong build at all. He also seemed to be going bald.

"Robbery," I said.

"Really, who did you rob?"

"No one," I said.

"No one? Then, how are you here?"

"Bad luck," I said.

"You're telling me," he said. "Hey listen, my name is White Snake. If you need anything, just let me know, okay?"

"Okay, thanks," I said.

I finished eating my breakfast, and I was headed back to lock down. I was concerned and afraid still, and I was uncertain of what to do if I were tested in a fight. I wouldn't know the first thing. I began to think that my cellmate had it out for me. The idea made me feel uncomfortable. However, I stuck it out, and I went back to my cell.

Max and I were together again. I began to write a letter to my little sister about Max. I also began to write a letter to my mom as well. I asked my mom for some money in the letter. I needed money for hygiene supplies and envelopes that had stamps on them.

"Bower!"

I heard my name clear this time, and I got up quickly from my desk to my door.

"Ya," I said.

199

"You're going to dental. Bring your identification card with you," he said.

The guard was tall with brown hair and brown glasses. I only had my white shirt on as I came out.

"Where is your khaki shirt at, Bower?"

"In my room," I said.

"Go back and get it."

I traveled back up the stairs, and headed to upper twenty-nine.

"Pop twenty-nine," he said.

I went inside my cell and grabbed my khaki shirt. On the way out, I began to button it up.

"Let's go, Bower. Hustle. Jesus, Bower, tuck your shirt in."

I tucked my shirt in, and I was in line with five other inmates. Three were black, and one was Mexican, and the other one was white. I followed the escort, and the escort was female. She was the guard taking us to dental. All of us waited near an elevator, and the elevator was near unit one. The elevator was shiny, and silver. It looked as if it only traveled a few floors. The prison didn't go very high, and it only had three floors, if that. We stayed as a group, and when the elevator rang, I was headed up with the group of six, six because of the escort. When we arrived, we went through two other doors. The waiting room for dental was small, and the room had wooden benches. The benches only seated about four people. The room was surrounded with thick glass in three directions. I had my identification card with me. By the time my name had been called, half an hour was already gone.

"Bower," she said.

"Here," I said.

"Let me see your identification."

I pulled out my identification card to where it was visible to her. A brief moment of silence took place.

"Okay, come with me," she said.

I followed the officer down the hall, which turned into a sharp left corner. There were nurses' stations surrounding the medical rooms. The officer led me to a large room with a doctor that had a white lab coat on, and he was wearing a pair of blue gloves.

"Come on down," he said.

I came down.

"Take a seat in this chair. We need to take some photos."

I sat in the seat, and I was placed in a leaning position. My legs were stretched outward as I was leaning back in the chair.

"The nurse needs you to open your mouth," he said. "She needs to swab your mouth for your DNA."

So I complied, and I opened my mouth. The doctor was touching my teeth, making me feel uncomfortable. He was sliding his fingers through my gums and in the back of my mouth. The nurse placed some film in my mouth after swabbing me and told me to bite down. The film was a gray looking color, and they exited briefly while taking photos from another room. This process lasted nearly ten minutes. I guess they were confused or something. When they were all done, no thank you was given. I was simply moved along to the next step. It took me extra strength to get out of the chair. I was in such an awkward position. I went back as instructed by the officer, and from there I was escorted back to the waiting room. As I waited, thoughts passed through my mind about my cellmate. I was still concerned for my safety.

I mean, I didn't know the guy. How was I to know if he were to attempt to kill me or not? I didn't, I didn't know at all. After we all grouped up again, the female escort took us back through the same way we came. I had a lot of thoughts rushing through my mind. So this time I went to the guard, and I felt I had to. I believed I had no options left. I wouldn't last in the cell, with this guy, for another night. Especially with his loud snoring.

"Hey officer, sir," I said. "Hey officer, I don't want to lock down."

I caught him off guard.

"What's that?"

"I said, I don't want to lock down, sir. Please can you keep me safe?"

The guard looked me up and down.

"Are you serious right now?"

"Yes," I said.

"Okay, put your hands behind your back," he said.

"Why?"

"Because we are sending you to segregation. That's why."

"Okay," I said.

As the blue suit placed the handcuffs on me, five other guards came to the unit.

"Okay, Bower, let's go. We're taking you next door," he said.

The five guards that showed up consisted of one female and four male guards. I was on my way to segregation where my next journey would begin. All I wanted to do was call my mom. Other inmates were looking my direction, whispering to one another. I was concerned by this, and the way the other inmates were acting seemed shady to me. As I was headed out the door, one of the inmates yelled out, "Snitch!"

 As the door shut behind me, the guards that were with me followed. I was escorted by two guards, as the other three branched off in different directions. I was escorted through the same hallway I came through from intake. I was headed to the Lincoln Correctional Center, from the Diagnostic Evaluation Center. The two guards who were with me were both white. One was tall and the other was short. The short one had red hair, and the tall one had blond hair, and both of them didn't wear glasses. And neither one of them was fat. I could tell they both lifted weights, and I figured that was their daily routine in life. We eventually passed a door, and that door led to another door. This door had a microphone and camera. After we gained access, we were led to another hallway. From there a gate laid before us, and when the guard unlocked the gate with a key, we were headed to a holding cell. Once we arrived at the holding cell, the taller guard removed my cuffs from my hands, and I was instructed to strip out. I was told to remove my boots, shirt, and pants. After I took my clothes off, I was instructed to lift my feet.

"I want to see the soles of your feet," he said.

Afterwards the guard continued.

"Bend over, spread your checks, and cough," he said.

"I have to do this again?"

"Just do it," he said.

I complied, and after the guard was finished, I was given back all my clothing except for my belt and my boots. I was told to step into the cell and have my

204

back turned to the guards. After I complied, the door was shut and locked behind me. I noticed a camera in the upper part of the cell, and it hovered right above the door. I looked through the window, and there I saw my boots laying on the floor. I got dressed in my boxers, pants, and shirt. I waited nearly an hour before the next set of officers came to attend to my prison needs. I was given a sack lunch for my meal, and it contained an orange, milk, and a ham sandwich. I saw a woman enter the unit to the holding cell, and the woman approached my door.

"Mr. Bower," she said. "I am Merry Faulson. I am the Lincoln Correctional Center Counselor."

"Okay, why are you talking to me?"

"Because I need to know if you feel like killing yourself."

"No, not at the moment," I said.

"Well, it's important that you be honest with me right now," she said.

"No, I don't feel like killing myself."

She had blond hair and blue eyes, and she was shorter than the average female. She also had a gap in between her teeth.

"Austin, I was asked to come speak to you from my supervisor," she said.

"Ya, and who is that?"

"Steven Manner."

"Don't know him," I said.

"Well, he says he knows you." He said he used to work with your father."

"Ya, my dad used to work here, so what?"

"He wants to help you," she said.

"Who wants to help me?"

"Steven does," she said.

"Okay, what kind of help?"

"You would go to the mental health unit," she said.

"What's that?"

"It's a unit for inmates with mental health needs," she said.

"Okay, when would I go?"

"You would go next week," she said.

"Okay, cool."

After that she left the holding area, and she shut the door behind her.

I waited about another hour, and then eventually the guards showed up to escort me.

"Okay, Bower, let's go," he said.

He began to unlock the hatch. The guard handed me my boots and my belt. I began to put my socks on, along with my boots and my belt.

"Okay Bower, I need you to place your hands through the hatch," he said.

I looked up in the corner and saw a black camera staring at me. After the guard placed the cuffs on me, he began to open the door. After the door was open, the guard instructed me to stand up, straight against the door. I did so, and the guard placed a belly chain around my waist. After the belly chain was tight against my waist, the guard applied ankle cuffs to my ankles; however, the cuffs wouldn't fit because they were too small. Yet, they were the biggest cuffs in the facility.

"Shit, Bower, what the fuck? Fuck, they won't even fit you. Hey, tell the sergeant that we are going to need bigger cuffs," he said.

The guard doing my restraints was talking to the guard behind him. The guard behind him was tall and large. The guard doing my restraints wasn't nearly as tall.

The guard doing my restraints was short and stocky. He looked as though he played football in his high school days.

"Fuck'n a, Bower, lose some fucking weight, would ya?"

I just stayed quiet through it all. I didn't say one word, and I just ignored it like it was nothing. The sergeant came down and had me looked over. He decided to use plastic cuffs for the time being. After the sergeant had me all ready to go, I was sent to the segregation unit.

Chapter 18 Segregation

Studies have proven that inmates with mental illness are 20 percent more likely to be assaulted by inmates who are not.

I was sent to the segregation unit, and I was placed in C-unit where all segregated inmates go. Inmates would come here for fights, and some came here if the inmate feared for his life. I was placed in cell three, upper tier, and it was my first time ever in segregation at this facility. I had been in segregation before in the county jail, but this was different, this was state time. This wasn't county jail time any more. The guards who hooked me up at my holding cell unchained me and placed me in my new cell. I was given no answers of what it would be like. I was just expected to figure that out all on my own.

Over time I learned that this place was evil, and it carried an evil presence to it too. I sat in my cell at my desk before I realized I needed to call my mom. I walked up to the door, and I began to yell for the case worker.

"I want my phone call," I said. "I want to call my mom!"

"I want my phone call to call my mommy!"

Another inmate began to mock me.

"Shut up!"

"No, you shut up," he said.

I figured that I would ignore him, and that I would continue to ask for my phone call.

"What do you want, Bower?" the case worker asked me, and he was standing at the base of the stairs.

"I want my phone call," I said.

"Okay, well you need to file a kite because you can't use the phone unless you're on the phone list," he said.

"Please I need to make my call."

"Just go lay down, Bower."

After he spoke, he walked back to the office that he came from.

"Hey, new guy!"

"Who's that?"

Someone was calling my name, and they were nearby.

"Hey, you can make a five minute phone call; it's policy," he said.

"Where is that voice coming from?"

"Get on your toilet," he said.

210

I looked around, and I stood on my toilet.

I noticed that I could speak through the ventilation system.

"I'm here," I said.

"Ya, you can make a five minute phone call," he said. "They have to let you."

"Really?"

"Ya, if they don't let you make it today," he said, "you won't be able to make it tomorrow."

"Why not?"

"Because they're crooked that way," he said. "Tell them you want your five minute notification phone call."

"Thanks."

"Hey, what's your name?"

"Holgon," he said.

"Okay, thanks Holgon."

"Don't sweat it," he said.

I took a look in my cell, and it was small and smelled of urine. I had a sink connected to my toilet, and my toilet had a toilet paper dispenser built inside of it. I had five kites laying on my desk, and I was given a state issued pen. I had a brown sack laying on my mattress. I opened the sack, and I took out the state issued deodorant and the state issued soap. I picked the soap up, and it didn't smell like normal soap. I also had a state issued toothbrush along with state issued toothpaste. Time seemed to go really slow in here. The moon was out, but I couldn't see it. I just knew that it was out because the sun was down. The case worker didn't bring me medication when the case workers passed out the meds. The case worker was going cell to cell.

"Hey sir, do you have my medication?"

"No, we don't have medication for you right now," he said.

He was large and tall, and he wore a blue shirt that read NDCS on the front of it. He also had a radio that clicked to his shirt from his pants. His radio was tucked into his pants, and the mouthpiece was up by his ear. He spoke in the mouthpiece by clicking a button whenever he wanted to talk. It was part of his radio, and I assumed he did it for his own convenience.

"What is your name?"

He came up to my door to see what I wanted.

"What did you ask me?"

"What is your name?"

He didn't hear me the first time.

"I'm Fondle," he said.

"Nice to meet you," I said.

212

"What is this, high school?"

"I don't understand," I said.

"Neither do I. Go lay down, and relax," he said.

"What about my phone call?"

"What about it?" he said.

"I'm supposed to have a five minute notification call," I said.

"Who told you that?"

"No one," I said. "But it is policy."

"What are you going to do, write a grievance?"

"Ya," I said. "Matter of fact, that is exactly what I will do."

"Here, let me get you a grievance form," he said.

"I want my phone call."

He picked up a grievance form from the white cabinet in the center of the day hall.

"Here you go, write your grievance, and make sure you spell my name right too."

He slid the grievance through my cell door while I was talking.

"I want my phone call," I said.

"You know what, fine, I will get you your phone call," he said. "Let me finish passing out medication, and then I will get you your phone call."

He was breathing heavy now, and I could tell that he wasn't happy. I watched him pass the medication out to all of the other inmates on my tier. He began to leave, and he took the phone with him.

"I want my phone call!"

He was headed down the stairs, and he stopped at the middle of the steps.

"You will get your call, Bower. You need to be patient," he said.

"Okay," I said.

I was standing at my door waiting for him to return. I waited ten minutes, and he began walking my direction from the other side of the unit. I could see him because there were so many windows built in my view of where I was housed. He had the phone in his left hand, and he was walking up the steps, and he met me at my cell.

"Here you go, Bower," he said.

He didn't sound too pleased either.

He began to unlock the hatch that was on the outside of my door. He then handed me the phone, and it was in hand held form. It was a black cordless phone, and it had clear buttons on it that lit up in orange when I dialed a number.

"You have five minutes," he said.

214

"Okay, thank you."

I thought of how important it was to call my mom. I began to dial the number, and it began giving me instructions.

"Please dial your inmate number," the phone said, and it was a female voice.

"Please dial your pen number, followed by your inmate number," the voice said.

"I don't have a pen number," I said.

I went to stand on to my toilet.

"Hey neighbor," I said. "How does this phone work?"

"You need to have money to make a phone call," he said.

"What? What if I have no money?"

"Then you're shit out of luck," he said.

"Really? How does my mom call me?"

"She doesn't," he said.

"What do you mean?"

"She can't call you," he said.

"Why?"

"That's just how it is," he said.

"Really?"

"Really," he said.

I had no use for the phone at this point because I had no money. I waited for the caseworker to return, so I could give the phone back. He soon returned, and I gave him the phone back through the hatch.

"Did you get through?"

"No," I said.

"Okay, if you're lying I will know," he said.

"I'm not lying," I said.

"Okay, but if you are I will know."

He took the phone, and he walked away from my cell door.

"Hey neighbor," I said.

"What?"

"How would he know if I made a call or not?"

"Because they record the phone calls here," he said.

"Really?"

"Really," he said. "Now no more questions for tonight."

I could hear irritation in his voice. It was late, so I decided to lay down and call it a night. I laid there looking at my ceiling. My ceiling was white and had lumps on it from the paint that didn't dry correctly. I finally fell asleep after tossing and turning throughout the night. The next day I had a really hard time accepting this as my life. I couldn't believe that this was where I was at. I hated it, and this was really prison. *It is freezing cold in here*, I thought to myself. The walls were white with concrete floors and a steel metal door. The cell was small, simply an eight by six cell block. There in the corner of my cell near the door was my toilet. I had a different view of things from my mattress. I also noticed that the hatch to my door was welded in. I could see the parts of melted metal, and it was a small square shape. It was also where food, laundry, books, and canteen items were passed through. The windows were very narrow, and they were side to side. However, that was the intent, so it would be less likely for an escape.

The bed I slept on was not a bed at all. In fact, it was a large plastic boat. I was able to move the boat and pick it up, or set it aside for cleaning purposes.

The walls seemed to be hollow, simply because other inmates next door would pound on the wall for their own entertainment. They did this to catch a rise out of another person's soul. It was sad really, and you would hear screams at night. Not just any normal screams; these were bloody murder screams. Yelling, crying, weeping, and sobbing. During the day in the ventilation system that hovered over the toilet I noticed other inmates would step onto the toilet, get into the vent, and begin telling others to kill themselves repeatably. Sometimes they got lucky and had a decent neighbor, and I was one of the lucky ones. I have seen a few affected by the provocation. One person almost succeeded in killing himself. It was while I was housed where I was now, and it was awful. The sad part was the guards would joke about it, and all the caseworkers would too. They would pass by my door laughing, as if it were nothing at all. Like a joke, or rather a sport, and it was so sad to watch.

It was December, and my cell was freezing cold and the days were long and dreadful. The days really drug out in solitary confinement because there was little to no noise at all. I didn't hear cars driving by or honking. And I most certainly didn't hear

people chatting, like they would in a coffee shop, by any means. I heard cries, rumors, and stories of inmates who were stabbed in the prison yard. Or people who were shot in the streets. I watched inmates who were mentally slower get teased and made fun of. I was one of them, and the word retard was used quite a bit.

"Hey retard, hey dumbass, kill yourself, bitch."

Those were only a few words out of the many used against me.

Then a response would arise from me, from a faint part of the unit.

"Leave me alone. I want to be left alone," I said.

Hardly a victim at all, especially in the eyes of society.

The more I reacted, the more inmates would step to their doors yelling.

"Kill yourself, you good for nothing piece of shit," they said.

"Ya, end your life, you dirt fuck."

As I continued to react, they would continue to yell. Then I would begin pounding on my cell door, and the pounding would be so loud it would wake everyone up out of their sleep. The guard would come down to the noise and check the unit to see what the problem was. Sometimes the guards would ignore it, and other times they would scream at me to shut my mouth.

"Shut your mouth, Bower!"

The guard would yell and point his finger at me.

"Shut your mouth, and go to bed," he said.

I was in my orange jumpsuit with silver buttons, and I would yell right back.

"No fuck that, these fuckers are telling me to kill myself. How am I expected to sleep when that is happening?"

The guard pondered the question, and then began to speak.

"It's not such a bad idea. Why don't you try it?"

"What?"

"Kill yourself, you good for nothing faggot," he said.

Then all hell broke out.

"You piece of shit blue suited bitch, fuck you!" I began to yell.

"You're the fucking faggot, not me," I said.

Then I pounded on my cell door, and as the third shift guard walked away, he acted as if he heard nothing at all. His walking away was a form of instigation. As I continued to pound, the comments from the other inmates continued as well.

"Kill yourself, you fat fuck fatty," they said.

"Ya, you good for nothing dick swallower!"

It took me nearly two hours for me to realize if I say nothing in return I can avoid them altogether. To them no answer means no fun, and I was that inmate providing entertainment. The next day would roll around, and the guards would be preparing the morning breakfast, which consisted of either toast and eggs or poorly cooked

pancakes. The unit would smell of urine and semen, not the best smell to wake up to.

The cell had a metal desk with a metal seat for eating purposes.

"Breakfast? Breakfast, Bower?"

I looked at the guard for a split second.

"Yes," I said.

The guard pulled out his keys and began to unlock the hatch. The guard then slammed down the hatch, passing through the tray of food. The food came in a yellow container, which had a lid to it. The container looked dirty with filth from past meals, most definitely unsanitary. The guard then went around in a L shape passing out the trays. There were two guards that were working, one was short and one was tall. The shorter one was bald, and the taller one had a widow's peak. The tall one was Gross, and the shorter one was Brutis. The coffee given to us was weak and bland. Very cold too, if I may add. After finishing breakfast, the guards would come by one by one picking up the trays. All that I heard were locks and keys rattling. There was also little conversation taking place during it all. It was my job to ask for items, and if I didn't ask I didn't receive. I had to ask for items such as toilet paper and kites, which kites are also known as request forms. Then during the morning hours the caseworkers would ask, one by one, if we wanted yard. In December the yard was extremely cold, and the guards would attempt to talk others out of going to yard. The guards had a come along chain set, which is a chain link that is connected to hand cuffs. They used this tool for safety measures, to keep order and control.

"Bower, do you want yard?"

221

"Yes," I said.

"It's cold outside, Bower. Are you sure you want to go out?"

"It beats being in this cell twenty-four seven," I said.

"Ya, but still it's cold out, and we're talking below zero," Brutis said.

I looked at both of them briefly, and they looked back at me in a moment of silence.

"Man, just take me outside," I said.

"You got it, but just so you know, if you go out, you will be staying out for the entire hour," Brutis said.

I stood up after the cuffs were complete around my hands.

"Okay."

The caseworkers opened the door to my cell, and we were on our way.

They both led me down the stairs that led to a lower level of stairs, and that led to the

door. Outside of that door contained three gated yards, which had barbwire at the top

of each fence. The yard fences carried three yard doors, and each yard door had a lock on it. The hatch was just like the indoor unit cell hatches. There were no weights and no pull up bars. It was simply a ten foot by six foot yard. Only walking space was granted in each yard. The correctional staff all went by their last names, and they never used their first names, except on odd occasions. The unit was full of killers, thieves, sex offenders, rapists, drug dealers, and more. The ones who received most of the negative attention were the sex offenders and baby killers. They were looked down upon as unworthy, and most sex offenders went to protective custody, otherwise known as the PC unit, which in the Lincoln Correctional Center is A-Unit. The days were mostly slow, and it was very important to attempt to stay busy. Unfortunately the only thing I could do was exercise my mind. It was very important to read and stay educated during the process of slow time. Books were of value in prison and in high demand. I went to yard thinking about my past and the days leading up to the robbery. Thinking back on the night that poor man was robbed was breathtaking. I had just graduated from high school, and I was young. I thought I knew everything, just like every twenty year old. Silly thinking back now, more like stupid. I trusted everyone with everything; moreover I was just too trusting I guess. I mean, I thought the friends I had hung around honestly cared for me. Little did I know, at the time I was wrong. It was the summer of 2009, and I had a few run-ins with the law enforcement here and there. Nothing prison worthy at the time, and I had thought stealing was cool and that I would be respected if I stole. I was convinced I was liked, moreover loved, for my many actions of loyalty for the many people in my life. Little did I know, these people would never steal for me. I was being used, I thought. After all, I had a lot of time to think about all these things behind bars, and I was a tool for their gain. However, at the time I was clueless, and I had no indication that this was how it was. Then a real devil came into my life; he was full blooded Native American. He claimed he was in a gang known as Lakota Theresa. He had tattoos all over his body, and he shared with me how he was from Omaha, Nebraska. I met him through a friend named Steven. This devil's name is Hawkboy, as you already know.

"What's good, Steven?"

I looked at Steven with honor.

"Not much, Austin," he said.

"Hey, I have someone I think you would like to meet," he said.

I was standing at his apartment door entrance, and the rail was rusted and the walkway was dirty. The walkway was littered with paper and trash. I could also see children's toys and a small tricycle that laid on the end of the walkway. It was pink with white handle bars.

"Come on in," Steven said.

I began to walk in, and I saw the carpet was brown with brown cabinets to match. There were two

224

people seated on the sofa, one of which was a young man, and the other was a elderly lady, who appeared to be in her sixties.

"Hawkboy, this is Austin; Austin, this is Hawkboy," Steven said.

Steven had a smile on his face too.

"What's good, man?"

Hawkboy looked me up and down.

"What's good?"

Hawkboy's voice was low, and it sounded like he didn't care.

I was back in my cell from yard now, and I was laying on my mattress thinking back. I wished that day had never happened, meeting Hawkboy, I thought. It really bothered me to think of how my life was caught up because I trusted the wrong person. My mother attempted to save me from all of that, but I was stubborn simply because I felt she had grown so distant from me. Oh how I wish I would have trusted my mother, especially now at this point in my life. I thought of how I trusted all of the wrong people.

The case manager came to my cell, and with him was the mental health counselor. The case manager unlocked my hatch and opened it.

"Hello, how are you doing, Austin?"

Merry was in good spirits.

"I am hanging in there," I said.

"Good," she said. "We are glad to hear it."

"So Austin," Kim said, "you will be going to the mental health unit. We will need you to sign some paperwork."

"Ya and you will like it there much better," Merry said.

"What do they have that's so good over there?"

"Many things," she said. "Canteen is better, and you get more freedom."

"Okay, so when do I go?"

"After all the paperwork is filed," she said. "You will most likely end up going in the next two to three days."

"Okay, go ahead and sign this form we have for you," Kim said.

I took the form and the pen, and I signed my name on the line, and I also signed my inmate number, *73223*.

"Okay, Austin, that is all we need for now," she said. "Oh, and I will no longer be your counselor, just so you know."

"Okay, thank you for telling me," I said.

I went into the back of my cell, and I laid down. I

would do the usual thing, such as eat my food and even read a book. I was in a one man cell, which made things easy for me. The days went by slowly, but I knew that I was leaving soon and to a different unit. So in a way that kept my spirits up, I went to the yard outside of my segregation unit, and I overheard two inmates speaking about a violent stabbing that happened in the Nebraska State Penitentiary, otherwise known as NSP. They both said the inmate who was stabbed to death wasn't even the initial target. I guess one inmate lied or something about his hood and convinced the inmate with the shank that it wasn't him. From what I gathered, it was all over a television. I guess an inmate stole another inmate's television, or something to that degree. I thought hearing that was crazy, and it really concerned me for my safety, due to other inmates who are out to get me. I was standing in the yard, and I asked one of the inmates a question.

"Hey man, I have a question for you," I said.

"Ya, what about?"

He was dark skinned and Mexican.

"Does the mental health unit have contact with the general population?"

"Ya, why? Are you scared to go back there?"

"Na, I'm not scared," I said.

"You better not be, or you will get eaten alive," he said.

"Ya right," I said.

"Okay, don't believe me," he said. "Fights happen all the time."

"Thanks for the heads up," I said.

After that small talk I said no more, and the guards cuffed me with the come along restraints, and I went back to my cell.

Chapter 19 The Mental Health Unit

Due to over crowding in the Nebraska Department of Corrections inmates with serious mental illness are not treated by mental health.

"Are you ready, Bower?" Lungs asked me.

He was tall and skinny with a short nose and brown hair. "Yes," I said.

"Okay then, let's get this show on the road," he said. "So what are you in for?"

"Robbery," I said.

"Robbery, really? You don't strike me as a robber," he said.

"Thanks, I guess."

"Well the good news is you don't have to wear chains because you are going to general population," he said.

Lungs opened my cell door, and he escorted me down the stairs and to the main segregation door. He unlocked the door after using his radio for clearance, and before I knew it, I was headed to the mental health unit. We both arrived at the D-Unit main door. The door read D-1. Down the hall was another main door, and that door read D-2. Both units were for mental health. Lungs opened the door, and I met four inmates right off the bat.

"We got a new guy today," Jerry said.

Jerry was tall and Indian. He had some tattoos on his left arm and on his neck.

"Hey new guy, I'm Jerry," he said. "What's your name?"

"I'm Austin," I said.

"What are you in for?"

"Robbery," I said.

"Ya, I'm in for burning a house down with the family inside while they were still alive," he said.

"Damn," I said. "That sounds crazy."

"Yep, and that is why I am here," he said.

"Hey, new guy, I'm Nick," Nick said. "But you can call me Info. I know the information on anyone and everyone."

I looked around the unit, and I saw many rails and stairs that led to cell doors. The cell doors to the unit had numbers above each door.

"Bower," Gordan said, "I'm caseworker Gordan."

He was short and had large arms and a strong build. His head was shaved, and he had a little facial hair.

"Let me show you your cell," he said. "You will be in lower 29."

He began walking me down the steps.

"You arrived while everyone was locking down," he said. "But you will still be able to come out for lunch. Lunch is in about twenty minutes."

I went into my cell and locked down for the next twenty minutes. My cell had a spring bed instead of a boat, and my cell had cabinets too. I had a large wooden desk, and it was a one man cell. The cell was a one man cell designed for transitioning inmates from segregation back into general population. I had no idea how long I would be in this cell for, a week, maybe two I thought. I was hoping that they would make it my final cell. I hated going cell to cell, and it was getting old really fast. I looked out my cell window, and I saw the caseworker opening a small box. Next thing I noticed was all the doors began to pop. My door made a clicking nose, and my neighbor's door did too. Everyone came out forming a group and began walking to the outer doors, which were on the lower level of the unit. So I just followed and went with everyone else. I heard chatter and lots of talking for being in prison and all. I noticed that things were not very segregated. Blacks talked to whites, and Mexicans spoke with Asians, and I noticed even a few whites claiming to be Native American. I was under the impression that prison was segregated and divided into groups. Obviously there was some mistake. That or the inmates were just fake. I remember watching documentaries about prison life and the thug life. This was nowhere near that. The unit, including me, walked to a gated fence, and the gate swung open to the big yard. We had to walk the big yard all the way to the chow hall, which was about a football field length away from the mini-compound.

"What's your name?"

He was a tall Indian man, and he had two missing front teeth. Navajo wasn't his real name, but that is what he went by.

"Austin," I said. "What's yours?"

"I'm Navajo," he said. "So Austin, what are you in for?"

"Robbery," I said.

"Okay, so you must be a tough guy," he said.

"No, I'm not," I said.

"You're not?"

"No," I said.

"Well, this place will test how tough you are," he said.

"I bet it will," I said.

"Are you getting smart with me?"

"No."

"That's what I thought," he said.

232

I tried to walk away from him, but he seemed to follow me, and I didn't like where this was going. I made it to the chow hall by entering a few doors that led to a long line. I noticed that there were about sixty to eighty inmates in line. I was five inmates ahead of Navajo. I felt safe for the moment. He tried to cut a few other inmates, and he was able to cut all the inmates in front of him. He was behind me now making me very uncomfortable.

"So Austin," he said, "Can you help me out with some money?"

I tried to ignore him, and I had no idea what to say.

"I don't know," I said. "I don't have a whole lot of money."

"Well when you do, can I get some of your money?"

"I don't have any money to give," I said.

"Okay, well once you do, I need about five hundred dollars," he said.

I continued in line and got further to the server.

"Think about it," Navajo said.

I grabbed my food tray, and I went to take a seat. I sat at the closest table to the front, which was where the guards were located. It made me feel a little safer. I was able to eat all my food, which consisted of two hot dogs and baked beans. I had some relish on the side for my hot dogs. I also noticed a large wall that

233

separated the kitchen from the chow hall. I also noticed a small square hole, where the dishwasher would receive dirty trays to clean the dishes. The chow hall was separated into sections. I guess Delta unit ate with Echo unit and Beta unit. I finished my meal and waited for the sergeant to call my group. I was the first one to the window, and I gave my dish to the dishwasher. I was headed back to my unit now, and I went straight to my cell. I was instructed to lock down, and so I did. There was a built-in television on the wall to my unit along with an exercise bike. Time seemed to go by at a much faster pace than it did in segregation. My counselor came up to my cell door. He was large, and he had a big waist. He had a bald spot on the top of his head, and he wore glasses.

"Mr. Bower," he said.

"I am Doctor Pukin."

He spoke in an odd way, I thought.

"You and me are going to meet in my office," he said. "Are you okay with that?"

"Yes," I said.

He had a key to my cell door, and he opened my door.

"Come with me, Mr. Bower," he said.

We both traveled up the stairs through the door to the main mental health office. Doctor Pukin led me to

234

his office. The main office was empty with no one inside. It was only Doctor Pukin and I.

"Take a seat please," he said.

"Okay," I said.

His office had a large white marker board and a large bookshelf. He also had a brown wooden desk, which had a computer resting at the top. His desk was covered with paperwork and large manilla folders. He had a large leather chair for himself, and near the door were two guest chairs.

"So, Mr. Bower, tell me about yourself," he said.

"Well, what do you want to know?"

"What is it that you think you have?"

"How do you mean?"

"Your mental health," he said.

"I know I have tourette's and autism," I said.

"Autism," he said. "You think you have autism?"

"Well I was diagnosed with autism when I was younger," I said.

"Really? I never would have thought you had autism. I have worked with individuals with tourette's before, and I can't tell that you have tourette's. But what do I know? I'm only a doctor."

At that he cracked a smile.

"So, Mr. Bower, has anyone on the unit caused you any problems yet?"

"Yet?" I asked.

"Yes," he said.

"Well, I don't know," I said.

"It's okay, you can trust me," he said. "Anyone at all?"

"Ya, I guess," I said.

"Who?"

"Well he calls himself Navajo," I said.

"Navajo, you say."

"Yes, Navajo."

"What did he do?"

"Well he asked me for money and things like that," I said.

"How much money?"

"Five hundred dollars."

"Wow, that's a lot of money."

"Ya I know, and I don't have five hundred dollars to give him," I said.

"Of course you don't. You know, I can have a word with him," he said, "if you want me to that is."

"No, that doesn't sound like a good plan," I said.

"Okay, Mr. Bower, let's get you back to your unit."

Doctor Pukin escorted me back to the unit, and I locked down in my cell.

"Okay, Austin, I will see you tomorrow."

For some reason Doctor Pukin gave me a bad vibe, and I didn't like it.

Chapter 20 The Fight

Those who practice Mental Health in the department of corrections do not look for symptoms of autism. More than two thirds of inmates treated for mental health have either Schizophrenia, or personality disorders.

I had been on Delta unit for about six days now, and I was doing fairly well. I had a small routine for myself, nothing big really. Just cleaning my cell and exercise during yard activities. I went to mental health groups with other inmates. The groups had two counselors and about seven inmates in full. The groups were held upstairs in a large cell, and I had only been to one of the groups so far. I thought it was awkward, if you want me to be honest. I hated it, and the other inmates seemed to be pretty stupid and unintelligent for the most part. Nevertheless, I tried to get along with them the best that I could. It was early morning, and everyone was getting ready for activities. Some were getting ready for work, and others were getting ready for the gym. The gym had two basketball courts inside, and there were speed bikes to exercise with. There was a non-activity section also, and that was where others played dominoes or cards. The gym was large and had staff offices built inside, along with a small locker room. I was still on the unit preparing to go to this gym all the inmates spoke of.

"Gym!"

Musk was a female caseworker in her mid fifties, and she was skinny and had long brown hair.

"If it's your day for gym, you need to line up," Musk said.

I was the first in line, and I waited near the front of the Delta unit door. After about five minutes, a few other inmates showed up for gym too. In total there were about eight inmates. That's when I had a bad feeling about something. Navajo lined up for gym about a minute before our departure. He had his white bandanna tied around his forehead, and he was looking right at me. Then Navajo broke the ice by hinting at his future plans for me.

"Austin," he said.

I said nothing in return.

"Why did you tell on me?"

I looked his direction.

"What are you talking about?"

I returned his question with a question.

"You know what I'm talking about," he said. "I'm talking about you and Doctor Pukin. Doctor Pukin told me everything."

At this I was worried because we were headed to the

239

gym, and I had a bad feeling something bad was going to happen.

"Let's go to gym, gentlemen," Musk said.

Musk escorted me and the other inmates to the gym, including Navajo. We walked a straight line down each hallway. There were boxes built into the wall at each corner hallway. Inside these boxes were cameras, and they were on twenty-four seven. As a group we went through double doors, and then from there we entered turnkey. At turnkey there was one metal detector and a wand search. After the wand search, there was a pat search. Each inmate went three at a time, and one at a time for the metal detector. Once we were all finished, we grouped up at the door, and we waited for everyone to finish. Once everyone was through, the turnkey guard pressed a button to open the gym door.

"Okay, you are all clear," she said.

The turnkey guard was black and had long hair with glasses. We entered the gym as a group, and we scattered our different ways throughout the gym. The gym was exactly as described to me. Two basketball hoops and an office along with an area for card games. The gym had oak floors and bleachers as well. The gym coordinator brought out the basketballs, and we began shooting hoops. Navajo was shooting behind me, and I could sense an off vibe about him. I had a feeling a fight was about to happen. I noticed two guards were occupying the gym at the time, and four of us were on the basketball court, Navajo being one of them. Navajo was still behind me. I felt his presence, and that's when he took his move. Navajo threw a basketball at my head, and I ducked right on time. He was in front of me now, and his hands were up. I took three steps back, and he took two steps forward. He swung once, and I wasn't expecting it. He hit me right in the front of my mouth, and blood soon followed. My hands were still down, and I wasn't ready for what was happening.

"Let's go, motherfucker," he said. "Fucking snitch. Let's go."

I turned, and I ran the opposite direction, and he chased close behind me. He caught up to me, and he began swinging at me some more, and I had no defense. He hit me in the mouth twice before the guards finally broke up the fight.

"That's what you get, bitch! You fucking rat! That's what you get," he yelled.

Navajo continued to repeat himself. I was placed in cuffs, as was Navajo, and we were both sent to segregation. During my walk blood was falling on my shirt and pants. I was in a lot of pain, and I needed medical attention.

"Okay, Bower, we have to take you to a holding cell," he said.

241

I waited in the holding cell for about an hour, and then I was escorted to the segregation unit. The guard was short with white hair and blue eyes. He looked to be in his mid-fifties. I was escorted through the hallway. Whenever I opened my mouth, I was in pain, and my teeth were very loose. This was the second time that I was hit in my mouth during lock up. The second time hurt much worse than the first time. I arrived to the segregation unit, and I was placed in an upper cell. The caseworker strip searched me and gave me an orange jumpsuit to wear. I sat in segregation for the next five days wondering what was going to happen with me. I met with the disciplinary court members, and they dropped all charges against me. In the misconduct report it had stated that I did not fight back, and so they dismissed all charges for a class one misconduct report. In a way I wish I had hit him back, but I didn't. Word got out that I ran from Navajo, and from there inmates played telephone. Some inmates would say I was raped by Navajo, and others said I was paying rent to Navajo. Neither of which was true, and even though I knew that, the other inmates didn't seem to care.

Chapter 21 The Hole again

Studies suggest that 16 percent of inmates in jails and prisons have a serious mental illness.

Hello, Austin," Merry said. "Hi," I said.

"We have some paperwork for you to sign," Kim said.

"Okay," I said.

"Well, Austin, they denied you to go back to the mental health unit," Merry said.

"Why?"

"That's why we are here today, Austin," Kim said.

"Why?"

"Well, we would like to send you to protective custody today," Kim said.

"No, I don't want to go back there," I said.

"Well, we feel that you wouldn't do well in general population," Merry said.

"Well then send me to the mental health unit," I said.

"We can't, Austin, because you don't have a severe

diagnosis," she said. "Plus you are unsafe in general population."

"I have autism," I said.

"You don't have autism, Austin," she said.

"Yes, I do."

"No, you don't," she said.

"Austin," Kim said, "can we please get you to sign this form?"

"No, I am not going back to protective custody," I said.

"Okay, well then we will have to place you on involuntary protective custody," Kim said.

"No, I want to go to the mental health unit," I said.

"Well, you can't," Merry said. "So are you going to sign the form or not, Austin?"

"No, I am not," I said.

"Okay," Kim said.

Kim shut the hatch to my cell, and both of them left my sight while walking down the steps. It was starting to get late in the evening and dinner was on it's way. I watched out my window as the food cart arrived. The guards began prepping the food trays. Once they were done, they started with my tier first.

"Bower, you want your dinner?"

"Yes, I want my dinner," I said.

"Well, here you go," he said.

The guard was standing at my door while unlocking my hatch.

I began to wonder why Merry thought that I didn't have autism. Merry told me that Steven wanted to send me there. She even spoke about how Steven knew my father. Was she pulling my leg? Was this some big joke? I grabbed the trays from the guard, and I looked in the food container. It was watered down pizza. How in the world does pizza have water in it? The bread was soggy and unworthy to be called pizza. I looked around and I became unsatisfied with my environment. So I took my sheets and pillowcase, and I flushed them down the toilet one by one. Eventually the toilet became plugged and the toilet water began to rise. The water began to poor out, seeping all over the concrete floor. The water would have ran for nearly five minutes before I was yelled at by the correctional staff.

"Hey, stop that now! Bower, you need to stop flushing that toilet right now!"

As I continued to flush my toilet, the staff surrounded my cell block.

"Bower, you need to stop that right now!"

I listen to no command given to me. I continued to flush, and flush the toilet I did. The guards got on their radios, and they called the sergeant to come to C-unit. The sergeant came down and expressed I would be moved to the control unit, which is a much more strict environment. The staff brought out a video camera and full body chains. I was threatened with chemical agents if I pulled any stunts while they were chaining me up. So I decided to go along with the program. I was emotional. In the back of my mind I thought I would be assaulted by numerous correctional staff. On the way to the control unit, I was brought to an elevator where the food cart went through. That's how they got food to the inmates in the control unit. The elevator smelt of stale fries along with stale vegetables. I was escorted by a female guard named Wax. Wax radioed the control unit staff, and they popped the first door. Wax had a second staff member helping her escort me, both of which were female. As I entered into the control unit, I noticed a large glass window. Behind that window were the correctional staff.

"What cell is Bower in?"

"Cell nine,"

"What cell?"

Wax couldn't hear the other officer very well. They were both speaking to each other through a thick glass next to a powerful looking gate. The gate had a large door connected to it.

"Cell nine!"

The control officer yelled louder this time. The guard was large and had black hair and large arms.

"Okay, got it," Wax said.

Wax was blond with thin hips and lack of a chest. She had blue eyes, and for a female she was tall. As I was escorted to my cell, I looked around and saw sixteen cell doors. I saw a few inmates peering out their windows. The windows were small squares and looked to be stained.

"Oh shit, oh shit, look what we got here," so it began.

I couldn't figure out what direction the noise was coming from.

"Looks like we got ourselves some fresh fucking meat."

"Hey, you fuckers see this?"

The inmates were talking to each other through their doors.

"Fresh meat, fresh meat," they chanted.

"Fresh meat, fresh meat," they continued.

"Hey guys, come and look at this fairy looking faggot right here," J.P Said.

I looked around, and all I saw were small squares windows, and they were surrounded by steel.

"I know who that is, J.P," Rodriguez said. "That's

the faggot who wrote a kite on me for selling drugs out of my cell."

I looked around, and I hesitated for a moment.

"Bullshit," I said. "What the fuck are you talking about?"

"Motherfucker, you know exactly what I am talking about," he said.

As the correctional staff were removing my chains, they were placing me in cell nine. The cell was cold and bitter. The cell was small, very small as a matter of fact. I hated it, every second of it. There were writings on the walls of gang language that read 'Bloods and Vice Lords united.'

There were all kinds of names written on the wall, such as *Mad Dog*, *J-six*, and *two guns*.

The wall was covered in obscenities. The walls were pale white and looked ugly. The cell had a fluorescent light on that was blinding.

No inmate had control of his own light whatsoever. When it was on, it was on, no questions asked. The same went for when it was off. An inmate named Lopez began to yell for me, and he spoke with profanities.

"Hey bitch, get up," Lopez said. "Bitch, what's your name? Fresh meat, hey bitch, I am talking to you."

His voice carried an accent, and it was easy to spot

he was Mexican.

"Hey J.P, what's that bitches name?"

"What? What did you say?"

"The new guy, what's his name?" the Mexican insisted.

"Who, cell nine?"

"Ya," Lopez said.

The Mexican sounded demanding.

"His name is Austin Bower," J.P said.

"Bower?"

"Yes, his name is Bower," he said.

"Okay thanks," Lopez said.

"Leave me alone," I said. "I'm not a bitch or a faggot! You fuckers need to leave me alone!"

"Leave me alone," they mocked.

"Leave me alone," they chanted.

They began to chant to one another.

"Whaaa, whaaa," they cried.

"I want my mommy," they mocked.

They began to make cries out loud to one another. I was standing at my door in ruins. My thoughts began to race over and over again. I began to pound on my cell door. My cell door had carvings in it, which had to have been done with a pen or a fingernail for that matter. My door echoed as I pounded on it repeatedly.

"Shut up, you fuckers!"

I was yelling so loud that I could feel my vein in my neck.

"You motherfuckers shut up!"

Tears began to roll down my face as I yelled back to their mocking and insubordinate behaviors. I was frustrated. I was mad. I was defeated and enraged. I was so enraged I began to cry out loud. My crying could be heard by the correctional staff. The door clicked to the bubble of where the correctional staff were located. All fell silent for a brief moment. The only noise that was heard were the boots of the guard. His boots made small bombing steps.

Thump, thump, thump was all you could hear. The guard finally arrived at my cell door.

"What seems to be the problem, Bower?"

He had a hint of arrogance in his voice.

"I want to die! I want to fucking die right now. Kill me please!"

The correctional officer was tall and large, with brown hair and blue eyes.

"Why do you want to die, Bower?"

"I can't handle it, that's why," I said.

250

"Please kill me now," I whispered.

I had tears rolling down my face.

Two other officers came to my cell, one skinny and one fat.

"What is the problem, Jackson?"

"Well Bower here wants us to kill him," he said. "Should we do it boys, should we kill him?"

He had a smile on his face.

"No, not for a piece of shit inmate like this, not worth it," he said.

They all began to laugh, all three of them. Laughing like it was a joke. I couldn't believe my eyes and ears.

"You better just lay down, Bower, and go to bed or something," he said. "Because I don't want to come out here again, do you understand?"

I looked away, and then I looked back.

"Can you make them stop instigating me please?"

"Bower, just ignore them and go to bed," he said.

I went to lay down, and it was quiet for a few minutes. Then out of nowhere they began talking again.

"Holy shit," Rodriguez said. "I mean holy shit, we got ourselves a snitch."

"Ya, that motherfucker is a snitch," Lopez said.

He was laughing while he said it too.

I tried to ignore them as much as I could, however it just seemed too difficult.

The noise of their laughter was haunting to me. Thoughts of the past began to entertain my

mind during their laughter. I felt so neglected by everyone. My thoughts started drowning out the noise. I started thinking about that night all over again. It was just like yesterday to me.

"We're gonna rob this guy," Hawkboy said.

"I don't want to do this," I said.

"Come on, don't be afraid. Have some balls and do this," Hawkboy said.

It was dark and warm on the Nebraskan summer night. The stars were shining and people were asleep. It had to be past midnight. During the day it was so busy with people driving to and from work, from and to school. The day finally ended, and everyone was winding down for the night. Very seldom people were outside, let alone driving.

"Come on, Austin. It will be all right," Hawkboy said.

I felt shocked, and I felt fear, as close as fear can get. I was so confused that I put my summer windbreaker on the ground. I placed it near some bushes at the bottom of the steps. I came up to the door, and Hawkboy was standing there just for a moment.

He positioned himself just right, and without further wait he kicked the door down. "Bang, bomb, crack."

The door flung open and Hawkboy was in instantaneously. I didn't move, and everything was in slow motion. I should have ran, but I didn't. So stupid, I thought.

"Give me the money! All of it," Hawkboy said while hitting the elderly man in the face repeatedly.

I felt my life pass through my fingertips. No coming back from this, I thought. My future was gone, and any dreams were too.

"Where's the fucking money?"

Blood was everywhere.

There was a small dog barking at my ankles. The dog was little and had white hair. "Bark, bark, bark," it said.

"Hawkboy, get off me," Chiko said.

The poor old man, I thought. I should have helped him. I didn't know how to fight though. Hawkboy would have turned on me and assaulted me instead.

"Give me the money," he said.

The fight went into the living room, and I attempted to grab Hawkboy to slam him. However, I missed and knocked Hawkboy and Chiko down to the

253

ground, and Hawkboy lost his shoe in the process.

The hatch was opened as I slowly arose from my prison mattress.

"Breakfast in bed, you can't beat it," Aims said. "It doesn't get no better than that."

Aims was old with white hair and white facial hair, and he was short and brittle. He had to be in his seventies or his eighties. Age got the best of him, and he appeared to be institutionalized himself.

"Juice, Bower?"

I looked through the window.

"Yes, please," I said.

"Please, who the fuck taught you manners? Had to be your boyfriend," Aims said.

I was upset now.

"I am not gay, you mean old man," I said.

The old man looked in my window. He wore glasses and his eyes were wide.

"I don't know," he said. "You look pretty gay to me."

"Get away from my door," I said.

"Okay, anything for you, sweetheart," Aims said.

I sat down to eat my breakfast, and the cereal tasted old.

We had two strips of turkey bacon, and I used my

sugar in my cereal. The tray was brown and thick, with four sections to it. The correctional staff went one by one picking up food trays. The day was slow, and it was shower day today. Monday, Wednesday, and Friday were all shower days. The sergeant would go to each cell number, one by one, for shower. The sergeant chose who would shower first, and then he would go in order from there. Steam would rise and fog up the mirrors as inmates showered. Two inmates showered before me, and then I followed.

"Run nine," Copley said.

My cell door popped for my shower, and I grabbed my shampoo and my conditioner. I had a bar of soap as well. I exchanged clothing and bedding items from the guards at the center cage. I received a new towel and wash cloth to the shower with. After that I went to the shower door. On my way to the shower I was insulted, mocked and teased by other inmates.

"Look at this ugly motherfucker right here," Lopez said.

"Fat stack faggot," J.P said.

"Hey, did you know this punk really reads the Bible?" Rodriguez said.

"Where's your God at now, faggot?"

I would ignore them and walk to the shower. The correctional staff would pop the shower door from the control panel. Showers were only fifteen minutes long. After fifteen minutes if you had shampoo in your hair, the guards didn't wait. They ran everything, water, food, canteen. You name it, they run it. As far as who walks the yard, well that was another story. Inmates ran the yard, mostly the lifers had that control.

Specifically lifers, murderers, killers. They said who stays, and they said who goes.

"Hey faggot, don't forget to shave your pussy too," Lopez said.

They all had names, every single one of them had a name. Brown, Kelly, Lopez, Mitchel, and Rodriguez. The worst out of the batch was Kogill, and he was bad. If anyone knew how to get you in a trap, it was him. Any day, every day. Especially on newcomers. He could convince anyone to fall for anything just to watch the sparks fly. The crazy part about it was the fact that he loved it. It was his entertainment, his joy, his masterpiece. He knew he was good at it too. The best.

He had convinced an intelligent convict that he was part of a powerful gang. He knew his stuff, and his words were practiced. He had a defense for everything too. I guess you could call him a jailhouse attorney.

"Ya, I roll with the eighty-eights," Kogill said.

"They call me White Tower," he said.

This guy was convinced too, and I couldn't believe it. The crazy thing is he knew people and their nicknames. This guy Kogill had a hell of a memory. I remember how he convinced this old guy that the correctional staff were poisoning his food. This guy

Chris bought the lie to such a degree that the correctional staff had to suit

up and use chemical agents to get his food tray back. I was astonished by his stupidity.

I am one to talk though. When I first met Kogill he had convinced me that staff had a piece of paper taped to their window.

"*Austin is a faggot,*" he said.

I believed it, and it was a lie from the devil himself. Nevertheless, I was convinced.

"Ya man, they have your name taped to the window," he said.

"It says *Austin is a Faggot.*"

Now I couldn't see the window from my cell, however Kogill could. I was just so convinced that I began to pound on my cell door, yelling and screaming. The correctional staff came to my door and asked me what the problem was. I was angry and frantic.

"I will kill you, all of you," I said.

 They looked puzzled.

"Bower, what is wrong with you?"

I grew even angrier.

"Take off that fucking note," I said. "The note on the fucking window right now, you motherfucking pieces of shit!"

"Bower, there is no note," Hill said.

"The fuck there isn't. Take it down now, you piece of shit!"

The guard was upset now.

"I'm not going to talk to you if you're going yell at me, Bower," Hill said.

Hill began to walk away.

"I am going to kill you, and I am going to kill myself!"

Hill came back momentarily.

"Did you state you were going to kill yourself, Bower?"

I looked at Hill through the small window. He was chunky with dark brown hair and brown eyes.

"Yes," I whispered.

"Okay, Bower, we are going to need your clothing and your pens," Hill said.

I looked surprised.

"Why?"

258

"You made self-harming threats," he said. "We have to take action when you say things like that. You will be moving to cell sixteen, the camera cell. You will have no clothing items, and you will have no mattress. Do you understand?"

He looked serious now.

"But why?"

"Because of your self-harming statements," he said.

I looked at him, and I took a deep breath.

"Why?"

"I already told you why, Bower," Hill said.

He went for his keys and unlocked the hatch.

"Give me your items, Bower."

I was confused.

"Seriously?"

"Yes, seriously," he said.

"If you don't comply, Bower, we will have to use chemical agents on you," he said.

I was upset and sad at the same time. Moreover, I was overwhelmed. I began to remove my clothing until I was butt naked. I handed over my clothing one by one, piece by piece. The guard shut the hatch, and he walked back to the control unit gate. He walked behind the cage, and then shut the gate, and as he shut the gate it echoed.

"Run nine," Hill said.

My door popped.

"Go straight ahead, Bower."

As I walked I felt played and manipulated when I saw no note on the window. I was in ruins. I couldn't believe how good Kogill had played me.

"Run sixteen," Hill said.

The door slowly popped open, and as I opened it I realized this would be my life for the next few months or even the next few years for that matter. I just wasn't sure about anything. How could I be in this situation? The cell was empty, and the walls were dirty with stains all over them. There was old food all over the floor and walls. The floor was sticky to my bare feet. The wall near my desk had a three prong outlet component system to it. It was for radio use only. That the guards even had control of. The desk was small and had a seat underneath it for a tight fit. The cell had a camera in it. The camera was in the upper right hand corner of the cell. The camera monitored any action that I did. All that I had in my cell was a piece of ground to lay on. No soft pillows and no soft mattress, which the correctional mattress is hardly soft anyways. I was sad, and I wanted to cry. So I did.

The days went by very uncomfortably.

I received a letter in the mail, and it had a money

order with it.

"Bower, I need you to sign for your money order," Echo said.

"Okay."

I received fifty dollars from my mother. Canteen was coming up, and I needed envelopes. I had to write someone about this injustice that was happening to me.

"Bower, you all right?"

"Man, why did you lie to me, Kogill?"

"Oh that, don't worry about that," Kogill said. "You'll be all right."

"Hey Kogill, I need some help," I said.

"What kind of help?"

"I need an attorney or something," I said.

"Ya, I can help you," he said. "But it will cost you."

"How much?"

"Five envelopes," he said.

"Okay, I can get that for you," I said.

"Okay, what do you want?"

"I want an address," I said.

"Okay, I can get you the ombudsman's address," he said.

"Whose the ombudsman?"

"Legal support," he said.

"Okay, ya I want that."

"Okay, get the envelopes, and then we will talk," he said.

"When will I get my stuff back, Kogill?"

"What stuff?"

"My clothes and my bunk."

"On Tuesdays," he said. "They review status on Tuesdays."

The security staff reviewed statuses such as mine on Tuesdays. *Shit, today is Tuesday*, I thought. *This can be a while for me. How can I survive this? Especially with others who mock me and instigate me?* I was dirty, and I could smell my own armpits. They smelled of old onions. My skin was pale white like a ghost. The mirror in my cell was scratched out by previous inmates who once lived in the cell that I now live in. My mind drifted back and forth from the past to the present. Little did I think of my future. I figured I would die where I lived. I felt worn out and beaten. I felt defeated and ignored. My voice meant something, I thought.

Nevertheless, I had no indication of how to use my voice. I had never been in a situation such as this one before. I had no idea how to channel my voice let alone the right way. I felt like an ant that had no purpose in life. The person next to me was crazier than I was, I thought. He would yell in the middle of the night waking me up from sleep. Great, I was sleep deprived and naked. How much worse can it get?

Worse it became indeed.

"Whack, crack, bang," the noise rang out in my ears.

"Boom!"

"Knock it off," I said.

The more I complained, the more he did it—imagine that.

"Hey, man, please stop," I said. "I really need to be able to sleep. Can you please stop?"

I had reason in my voice when I asked.

The tears began to flow down my face as I whispered.

"Please stop," I said. "Please."

While rocking back and forth on the cement floor, all I could think about was my mom and how she would come and save me. How my mom would come and save the day.

"Mom, please help me," I whispered. "Mom, I need you now more than ever. Please, Mom, save me from all of this madness."

263

I continued swaying back and forth on the cement floor while my back lay against the back wall of my cell. I would eventually sway myself to sleep regardless of the noise caused by my neighbor.

The loud intrusion it was, the ventilation system to the control unit was connected to each cell. Speaking through them was an easy task to accomplish.

You could have full conversations with other inmates through the ventilation system.

The nights were long at times, sometimes longer than the days. The days were long too, and regardless of how long they were, I hated it. I hated every second of it. I hated the other inmates, and they hated me.

I hated the correctional center staff, and they hated me, which made the environment much more stressful. Life in general was stressful, especially in prison. In

chains, bound and tied up in a box. There was violence everywhere. Stabbings were

spoken of, fights were spoken of. It didn't seem to end, and I wanted out. Earlier in the day the inmate in cell ten was moved. His name was Maxwell. His name reminded me of Maxwell coffee. Kogill was still at his old schemes attempting to mess with other inmates.

"Marcus, pack your shit. You're moving to ten," Copley said.

I was confused. I had put up with Marcus for the past few weeks, and yet he moved before me. I was often quiet and often respectful. How could this be?

I was angry, and it just made no sense, I thought.

It made no sense at all! I suffer for two weeks, and they favor this punk?

What kind of shit is this?

"Well, well, well," Kogill said. "Tisk, tisk tisk. You see, Bower? They hate you. But I don't, Bower. I love you."

The door to the center gate popped open, and Copley stepped out.

"Bower, come and grab your mattress and boat," he said. "We will leave it here for you to pick up."

The sergeant carried my mattress and my bunk to the outside of my cell.

"Run sixteen," Copley said.

My door popped, and I grabbed my mattress and my boat.

"Do I get to have my sheets and clothing too?"

"No, you were only granted those two items for now," he said.

I brought my belongings into my cell, and I shut my cell door behind me. Hours upon hours were spent in my cell doing nothing but writing. Writing was all

265

that I did. I read books when the book cart came around. Not much of a book cart though. Usually they had only six to seven books to read. On some days the books were really good ones, can't put down kind of material, and the books ranged between great or just plain horrible. Thinking was also another thing that you had to do all day. Not because you wanted to, rather because that's all there was to do. When I wasn't reading or writing, I was thinking. I was thinking all the time. I was still in cell sixteen, and I wanted out. I wrote the ombudsman a letter telling him I planned to kill myself. I paid Kogill five envelopes for the address, and I also bought phone time. I bought five units of phone time, which meant I spent twelve dollars and fifty cents on phone time, which equaled up to forty-five minutes on the phone.

"Bower, you want your phone call?"

She was white with red hair.

"Ya," I said. "I want to call my mom."

"I don't care who you want to call," she said.

The guard placed the phone up to my hatch. This phone was different than the one on

C-unit. This phone was on wheels, and it had a cord to it. It looked just like a pay phone at a phone booth. I dialed the number that I wanted to call. The voice asked me to punch in my inmate number and my pen number. The phone began to ring.

266

"Hello," my mom said.

"Mom," I said.

We were both interrupted by the female voice on the phone.

"You have a phone call from an inmate in the Lincoln Correctional Center," the voice said.

My mom accepted the call.

"Mom," I said.

"Hi honey," she said.

"Mom, they have me in the control unit, and they are treating me bad," I said. "They are saying I don't have autism, Mom. You know that I do."

"Yes, I know, and I sent paperwork to the mental health worker there," she said.

"You did?"

"Yes, I am also involved with the ombudsman's office, sweetie."

"You are, Mom?"

"Yes, I am, honey," she said.

"Mom, I feel like killing myself because this place is so bad," I said.

"I know, just stay strong," she said.

"Okay, Mom."

267

"It will be okay," she said. "Give it over to God."

"Okay, Mom," I said.

"Pray about it," she said.

"Okay."

"You have one minute remaining," the voice said.

"We only have one minute left, Mom," I said.

"I know, I heard."

"Okay, Mom, I love you."

"I love you too," she said.

After that I hung up the phone.

"Are you all done, Bower?"

"Ya," I said.

The guard took the phone and shut the hatch to the door. She walked the phone to the next inmate signed up on the phone list. I thought that was a short phone call. I couldn't believe it was only fifteen minutes. It didn't feel like fifteen minutes, I thought. I decided to write a kite to the mental health staff. I would write kites asking to be let out. I would also write the mental health doctors to give me treatment, and they would come back with inexcusable responses. Their response often refereed back to my behavior and that I had to manage well, and then they would talk about it. I learned fast that the correctional staff took very little responsibility, yet they would tell us we need to learn a thing or two about responsibility. Hypocritical, I thought. I was losing my mind, and I felt like breaking. I began to pound my head against the wall over and over again. I saw blood coming from the front of my head. I would leave blood prints on the wall, and it looked ugly. Eventually a scab grew over my forehead. I was in the control unit when the counselor decided to make her rounds, It was Merry.

"Merry," I said. "I knew you would come down to see me."

"Ya, I heard you were hitting your head," she said.

"Ya, I want to die."

"Do you have a plan?"

"Ya, I'm going to hit my head until I give myself a concussion," I said. "Then when I go to sleep I won't wake up."

"Okay, well you know we will probably have to send you to the hospital," she said.

"I don't care," I said.

"Well the Ombudsman does, and they got your letter. So we will be sending you to the diagnostic evaluation center."

"They got my letter I wrote them?"

"Ya, and they weren't happy with you either," she said.

269

"I didn't do anything wrong though," I said.

"Ya, you did."

"What?"

"You said we weren't helping you," she said.

"You're not. You call keeping me in solitary confinement helping me? This is not helping me," I said.

"Austin, you are the most seen inmate in this facility," she said.

"That's a lie, and you know it. You guys don't even treat my diagnosis.

"Is this going to be about your autism again, Austin? You don't even have autism, Austin," she said.

"You're telling me that all my past doctors are liars then?"

"No, what I am telling you is that you don't have autism at all," she said.

"Yes, I do. How would you even know anyway? You're not even a doctor. My mother even gave you the paperwork," I said.

"Your mother is wrong, Austin," she said.

"No, she is not," I responded.

"You know what, this conversation is over," she said. "You will be going next door."

After that Merry walked away and shut the gate behind her. The guards came to my cell about an hour later with full body chains, and they cuffed me and sent me to the diagnostic evaluation center.

Chapter 22 The Metal Table

The Nebraska Department of Corrections has a 31.4 population percentage of inmates who have been diagnosed with at least one or more mental health diagnosis.

I arrived at the diagnostic evaluation center, and it had fourteen cells all included. There was a control cage to the left and a black cage in the back. The black cage had an exercise bike and a television, along with a book cart full of books. It had a collection of old westerns. The unit had cameras in it. Some of the cells had cameras installed in them as well. In the front of the hospital was a shower and bathroom combination. The guards escorted me to a cell that had a metal table for a bed. The bed looked hard and uncomfortable. There were straps on all four corners of the bed.

"Where is Bower going?"

She was female with brown hair and a long nose.

"He is going into the full bed restraints," James said.

James was tall and white with a beard.

"What? I don't want to go on that bed," I said.

I began to refuse.

"You're going on the bed, Bower," James said.

"No," I said.

"We are going to need more staff down here," James said.

The female officer got on her radio and began asking for back up.

"Copy," the radio replied.

The radio beeped and more guards began to show up, surrounding me in seconds.

"Get him on the bed," James said.

The guards held my arms and my legs, and they began to unchain me. Once they had me unchained, one of the guards held my neck and the other three held my arms and my legs. I was resisting, and they were holding me firmly so I couldn't break free.

"Get him on his back," James said.

"No," I said. "Please don't do this. Please don't."

"Move his feet over to the left," James said.

The guards had my back fully on the metal slab now. They held my legs and my arms on the bed. One of the guards had my head in the palms of his hands. They were holding me still. I was afraid the guard was going to twist my neck.

"No, let go of me," I said.

"Hold him down," James said.

273

"We got him; he isn't going nowhere," said the officer.

While he was holding my head in one spot, I could feel the pressure from his fingertips.

"No, let go of me," I said.

The guards began cuffing me to the bed. They began with my hands, and then they held my limbs in place. Then they moved to my feet.

"Let go, please," I said. "I will be good. I won't write any more letters. I want my mom."

"I want my mommy," James mocked. "Can you hear yourself right now?"

The guards had me tied down, and cuffed. They began to leave one by one. The metal bed was painful to my back, and I was in pain. I could feel my hands losing circulation from the restraints.

"Help, I can't feel my hands," I cried. "Help!"

I was screaming and yelling now.

"Help me!" I said.

I was left on this metal table all alone, and the guards came back into the cell. They had a long strap, and they began hooking it up to the bed. They took the strap and they laced it underneath my arms like a weave. The strap went over my chest, and it forced both of my arms to lift up off of the bed. The bed was a metal box.

"Help me," I said. "Please let me off of this table."

I was in pain, and I was suffering. I couldn't believe the pain I felt in both of my arms.

"Help me, please," I cried.

The guard came into my cell.

"You need to shut up, Bower," he said. "We have patients who are trying to sleep."

"Fuck you," I said.

"Let me up," I cried.

"No," he replied.

He walked out of the cell and shut the door behind him. I was stuck laying on this metal table, and it was cold. I was facing the window that peered to the outside. I had a toilet in my cell, and it was near my head. There was also a camera in the cell, and it was right above me.

"Help me," I said.

No one came to my rescue, and I was left on this bed to die. My upper back was thrusting in pain, and my neck was hurting. The pain felt like a burning sensation.

"I have to use the bathroom," I said. "Please, I have to use the toilet."

I continued my attempt by yelling.

"I need to use the bathroom!" I yelled.

275

No one came to my aid. I had to go poop really bad, and I also needed to urinate.

"Hey, can you please let me up to use the bathroom?"

No one came to let me up to use the bathroom. This is great, I thought, just great. I needed to use the bathroom, and they wouldn't let me. I couldn't believe it because there was a toilet in my cell right next to me.

"Fine, you won't let me use the bathroom, well then I will just have to go pee on the floor."

Still no one came to my cell. I had been yelling for over an hour now. I began to slowly pull down my pants, and I finally got my pants down with my hands forced to my sides. I eventually got them down far enough to lean to the side and go pee.

"I'm peeing," I said. "I am peeing all over the floor."

Still no one came to the cell to check on me. I turned back into the frame, and I had pee all over my leg and my stomach. I had to go poop too, and I had no idea how I was going to be able to do that. I turned my body to my side the best that I could, and I leaned my ass over the edge of the metal slab, and I began to go poop.

"I am going poop," I said.

I could feel the poop slide down the side of my leg and off to the side of the bed.

"I went poop," I said.

I laid back into place and waited for staff to come. I had feces all over my ass. The staff began making their rounds while I was lying in my own bodily fluids. James began to unlock my cell door.

"God, what is that smell?"

"You wouldn't let me use the bathroom," I said. "You left me with no choice. I was yelling for an hour."

"Jesus Christ, Bower," he said.

He was covering his nose and mouth while he was talking.

"You should of let me use the toilet," I said.

James looked at me.

"You can lay in your own shit and piss now," he said.

"I need a shower though."

"You should've thought about that before you did what you did," he said.

"I had no choice though," I said.

James began to lock the door as he left the cell.

"Hey wait," I said. "Please! Don't leave me like this, please!"

The guard was gone now. It was nearing dinnertime, and I was too unclean to eat any food. I could hear the guard getting the food cart ready. He began to pass out the food to the other inmates. I noticed that I was the last one to be fed.

"Bower, we have your food," James said. "How do we do this?"

He was speaking to the nurse, and the nurse had on a blue uniform and white running shoes.

"Undo one of his hands, and he can use his fingers to eat his food," she said.

"Okay," he agreed.

The guard began to untie my left arm with his key.

"Okay, Bower, eat up," he said.

There were still feces on the floor and urine on my leg.

"What are you going to do about my shower?"

The guard looked at me with a mean look.

"You aren't getting a shower tonight," he said.

"Why not?"

"Just eat your food," he said.

"I can't. The belt over my chest won't let me," I said.

"What in the hell, Bower," James said.

He began to untie the belt that went over my chest and under my arms. I sat there eating my food, and I dropped some of it on my lap. I was eating hamburger helper with my fingers. I ate for about five minutes.

"I need some water," I said.

"You're not getting any water," he said.

"I need some though."

"Well too bad."

"Okay, that's how it is?"

"Ya, that's how it is," he said. "Now eat your food."

"I'm all done."

"Great."

He seemed irritated, and after I finished, James placed my hand back into the restraint, and he placed the strap back over my arm.

"No, please," I said. "I don't want that strap over my chest. No, please!"

"Too bad, Bower, it needs to go back on," he said.

James placed the strap back under my arms, and then they both prepared to leave.

Then both James and the nurse were gone, and James shut the door behind him. I was laying in the full bed restraints overnight, and I was in pain.

"Help," I said. "Please let me out of this! Someone please!"

No one came to my rescue. I was stuck in these full bed restraints, and no one cared. I still hadn't showered, and a shower sounded good right about now. My hands were dirty from the hamburger helper.

"Help," I said.

"Shut up!"

An inmate began to yell at me, and I could tell he was nearby.

"No, you shut up," I said. "I need someone to help me!"

The nurse came up to my window. He was black, and he was wearing a stocking cap.

"What do you want?"

He was smiling.

"Why are you smiling?"

"I'm not smiling," he said.

"Yes, you are," I said.

"No, I am not."

The nurse turned the light on to my cell, and he really wasn't smiling. I was blown away by this, and I felt an evil presence nearing me.

"Can you please let me up?"

"No, that's not up to me," he said.

"Who's it up to then?"

"All I know it's not up to me," he said.

"Please," I said.

I was in pain, and my back felt like it was caving in. The nurse turned the light off and walked away.

"Come back," I said.

"Come back!" I began to scream.

No one returned, and I was left there overnight. The next day came, and they still hadn't let me off of the restraint table. Time felt like it was slipping through my fingertips. I had no idea how many days had gone by. I was thinking three maybe four, but I was unsure. The same routine happened where the guard would unlock my left arm to let me eat. Then he would place my arm back in the restraint. The nurse would come by and check my vitals to make sure I wasn't dying. I felt like I was dying mentally and emotionally. I was dying, and I knew it. This experience was making me insane. It was driving me crazy, and it was taking me away from reality.

"Help me," I said. "I want to be let up."

I still hadn't showered, and I was losing my grip on everything. The nights went by with me being left on the metal table, and I wasn't even thought about. I lost all sense of time, and the clock meant nothing to me.

"Let me up," I said.

I looked out the window, and it was dark outside. The cell door began to open, and I could hear keys behind me.

"Mr. Bower," Evens said. "I am counselor Evens. Man, you look like shit," he said.

He had a Huskers baseball cap on. He was wearing a red t-shirt and blue jeans.

"I can't believe they called me out here for you," he said. "Look at you, you look like a piece of shit. Man, you are a waste of my time. You need to do what they want you to do and shut your mouth. I'm leaving."

"No wait, please," I said.

"What?"

"Please have me let up," I said.

"No, you're a waste of time."

At that he was gone, and the guard began to lock the cell door back up. His words repeated in my head over and over again. I was so bothered by his words to the point that if I could kill myself I would. I felt like dying, and I knew I was dead to these guards and mental health staff, and If I could kill them I would. If I had a gun right then and they let me off of that table right then, I would gun them down one by one. I never had the desire to kill someone like I did right then. I wanted to murder them one by one. One at a time, and just shoot them dead. Even stabbing them would be good enough.

"Help me," I said.

I was on this table for over the period a person should be, and I hadn't had a shower either. I was going crazy, and I was losing my mind.

"I'm gonna kill you fuckers," I said. "I am going to kill you all one by one!"

"I need some water, please," I asked.

My lips were dry and my throat was sore from crying for help. I had no idea what time it was. All I knew was the guards would be in soon to feed me. I lost track of how many meals I had, and I lost count of my days. My mind would wander in and out. I was in pain throughout my entire body. I felt a shooting pain in my neck and in my arms as well. I looked at my arms, and I noticed that I had bruises on them. I had big brown bruises.

"Help me," I said. "Help me, please!"

It was dark outside, and I saw through the window. I heard a noise coming towards my cell, and it was the guards.

"Thank God," I said. "Are you here to let me up? Thank you."

I noticed there were four officers, and the officers took my hands out of the restraints. Then they took my legs out of the restraints.

283

"Okay, Bower, let's turn you over," Micky said.

"What? No, please don't. No, please, don't do this!"

All four of them turned me around, and I was facing the metal slab with my face now.

"No please," I said.

I tried to fight, but I was too weak.

"Bower, you are going back into the restraints," Micky said.

"No," I said. "Please, not like this. Not like this, please."

Tears were falling down my face. I was now facing the table. My face was smothered by the metal slab, and my back was facing the ceiling.

"Please let me up," I said.

They began to leave after they restrained me. It became hard for me to breathe because my stomach had pressure from the table.

"Please don't go," I said. "Please come back."

I was crying and weeping. I could no longer see out the window, and I still hadn't showered yet, and my cell smelled horrific.

"I have to go pee, please," I said.

I couldn't see anyone.

"Please, I have to go pee."

I waited about an hour for a response.

"You have to go pee?"

"Yes," I said.

"Well, I can't come in there," he said.

"Please," I said.

"You are on your own."

"No, please come back!" I cried.

I laid there, and I held in my urine as long as I could. Then I was left without a choice, and I peed all over my lap. I could feel the urine, and it was warm and the smell was awful.

"Please let me up," I said.

No one ever came to my rescue, and I stayed in this position for days. I just laid there, and no one seemed to care at all.

"Help me," I said.

I began to fall asleep. My eyes were heavy and my body was sore. I couldn't believe this was happening to me.

"Jesus, I need you right now," I prayed. "Jesus, these men and women are evil."

I began to pray to Jesus.

"These guards have wicked hearts," I prayed. "Jesus, save me from this place please. Have mercy on their souls, Jesus, please."

I was crying, and I could taste my tears running into my mouth.

"Jesus, please help me through this," I said.

The next day the guards came into my cell, and they turned me back to a normal position. I was facing upwards now, and my back was back on the metal slab. My hands and feet were back in restraints facing up. Merry Faulson came into my cell, and she was in the presence of two officers.

"Mr. Bower, we plan to let you out as long as you stop yelling," she said.

"We will untie your left hand and your right foot," she said. "You will stay in two restraints until we feel you are ready to be let up. Do you understand?"

"Yes, I understand," I said.

The officer removed two restraints out of the four, and my left hand and my right foot were unrestrained. I laid there in pain and brokenness. I felt sorrow, and I felt defeated in many ways. I couldn't believe it was almost over. After more than three weeks of being tied down to this metal table, it was almost over. The pain and suffering of what my body felt. I laid there quietly, and I didn't make a sound. I kept my mouth shut for the next five hours. I knew that if I kept quiet it would soon be over. I hope they weren't lying to me, I thought. I really hoped they were feeding me the truth. I wanted revenge, and I wanted to kill them for what they did to me.

"Mr. Bower, we're letting you up now," Merry said.

"You can take a shower, and then we are sending you back to the control unit."

"Okay," I said, and they let me up.

Chapter 23 Defeated

The Centers for Disease Control and Prevention (CDC) indicate that approximately 1 in 68 American Children are on the autism spectrum.

I was back in cell sixteen broken and defeated. I felt like I was dead, and even my arms were limp. I lost all track of reason, and I no longer knew what reason was. I had no sense for it. All I could think about was getting out and shooting these fuckers to death. That was my plan, and it seemed pretty good to me too. I kept reading my scripture in the book of Romans, and I tried to understand. However, there was nothing to understand. They were evil, plain and simple. No further explanation needed, and something needed to be done, and it needed to be done by me. One good thing I had was my Bible, and they even tried to keep that from me. I had the first amendment that safe guarded that right of mine. All I did was read; I mean what else could I do?

The officer was going around with the medication cart and supplies. He had short hair and a long nose. His blue outfit made him look worse with his long nose. I thought he was ugly if you were to ask me. I'm sure he thought the same way about me too.

"Do you want your meds, Bower?"

"No," I said.

I began to refuse my medication.

"Are you sure you don't want your medication?"

He was asking me like I was a child.

"No motherfucker, can't you take no for an answer?" I said.

At that he shut my hatch, and he was gone.

"Fuck," I whispered.

I was in my cell with nothing. No boat, no mattress, and no clothing.

I was in my cell with absolutely nothing.

"Fuck this shit," I said.

"Fuck this shit!"

I was angry and extremely upset. These fuckers stole my innocence, I thought. These fuckers stole my dignity.

"Fuck you, motherfuckers," I said.

"Fuck you, motherfuckers," Lopez mocked.

"Shut up," I said. "Shut the fuck up!"

I was in my own hell, and the prison administration designed it to be that way. I would write request forms to the unit administrator and the unit manager, and they would tell me to work with the mental health team. So I would write the mental health team, and they would refer me to write the unit staff, and on and on it went. I would receive no answers to my current situation. They would always bring up my behavior and use me as their scapegoat. I began to realize this is how it would be for the remainder of my sentence. I realized mental health didn't want to help me, and neither did this administration. I was on my own, and I knew it too. Throughout my sentence I have lost two years of good time from verbal threats and petty misconduct reports, all of which accumulated to two years, and I would have to earn those two years back some how. I was broken without a doubt.

Chapter 24 Disciplinary Court

The (CDC) has estimated that 1 in 42 boys, and 1 in 189 girls are diagnosed with autism in the US.

T he state court process for when matters dealt with good time were split up into sections. Sections that could cost thirty days loss of good time and six months loss of good time. Even one year loss of good time. Sections were things such as verbal threats or physical altercations, and even masturbation could result in a loss of good time. The disciplinary court committee was based off of fractions and codes. The officers who did the committee were Chairmember Grades and officer Maxonn, both of which conducted the operating process of paperwork filed through a higher form of government, which would impact the inmate depending on his charges against him. The committee was stationed in the bottom of the control unit. The committee was prepping to set up against me as an inmate. They had to hook up cords and a computer with a microphone. Maxonn came out through the gate, and he approached my cell. Maxonn was white, and short, and he was no bigger than a high school freshmen.

"Bower, do you wish to be present for your

committee hiring today?"

"Yes," I said.

"Okay then, we will need to hook you up. Before we do, I want to go over a few things with you. So do you know your charges pending?"

"No," I said.

"Okay, a count two is pending of verbal threats and a count three of disrupting an officer's duties," he said.

"You had twenty-three other counts we had to dismiss," he said, "on the findings that the counts are seven days past the warranted statute of limitation. So we won't charge you with those. But we have two we are charging you with. Now that you are aware, are you ready for court?"

"Yes," I said.

"Great, we will get you hooked up then," he said.

The sergeant brought out chain restraints, and following him was the officer under the sergeant's supervision.

"Okay, let's get you chained up," Copley said.

The sergeant began to hook me up in handcuffs, and afterwards he had my door opened. He did the belly chain and my leg irons as well.

"Okay, Bower, let's move out," he said.

They led me to the office stationed in the control

292

unit, where my court was being held.

"Take a seat," Copley said.

"Okay, let's get started," Grades said.

He was black with a tight haircut, and he had a white dress shirt on and a pair of slacks. His eyes were brown, and his nose was flat.

"I am leading chairmember Michael Grades, and along with me is my ranking chair officer, Tim Maxonn," Grades said. "This court is being held today in purpose for inmate *Bower 73223*. State your name and number for the record."

"Austin Bower, 73223," I said.

"Very good," he said. "I have inmate Bower present. The first finding is count two verbal threats," he said.

"The report is as follows, 'I officer James of the diagnostic evaluation center, at approximately one-thirty in the afternoon, watched inmate Bower, 73223, threaten staff that he was going to kill them.' How do you plea, Mr. Bower?"

"Not guilty," I said. "I didn't say I was going to kill anyone."

"Okay, you may step out, and we will call you back when we are ready for you," he said.

The sergeant escorted me to the hallway and shut the door behind us. I was standing with the sergeant and the officer under the sergeant's supervision.

"Did you do it, Bower?"

"No," I said.

"That's hard to believe," Copley said.

"I didn't do it."

"Well, they will have the verdict in a few minutes," he said.

"Okay, he can come back in," Maxonn said.

I entered the office, and Grades began to speak after I sat down.

"In the findings of count two, we find inmate Bower guilty of verbal threats," he said.

"You will lose three months of good time for your behavior."

"Wow," I said.

"Let me finish," Grades said.

He was upset after I interrupted him during his testimony.

"You can earn this good time back with good behavior after six months of no misconduct reports," he said.

He kept looking at his computer screen, and he began to move to the next section of my misconduct report.

"I am leading chairmember Grades, and next to me is ranking chair officer Maxonn. We are here today for

294

the purpose of inmate Bower 73223. State your name and number for the record."

"Austin Bower, 73223," I said.

"Very good," he said. "This is a count three misconduct report. I will have to refer you to unit disciplinary court. This count three of interfering with an officer's duties will be held in the next seven days of unit disciplinary court. This closes our hearing for today. I am officer Grades signing out."

At that moment I was led back to my cell. Sergeant Copley was an unpleasant person to be around. I thought if he acted this way here, then he probably acted this way with his family. I wouldn't be surprised if he yelled at his wife the same way he yelled at some of us inmates. I was escorted back to my cell from the office, and I dreaded the walk back, knowing that I would stay for another three months. I mean, I already have two years I need to earn back. Something needed to change, and I hoped things started changing soon.

Chapter 25 Visiting

In 2001 Human Rights Watch estimated that at least 140,000 inmates had been raped while incarcerated in the united states by other inmates, and correctional officers.

"Bower, you have a visitor," Lanes said.

He was short and fat with long brown hair.

"So who is here to see you?"

"I don't know," I said.

I was given my khaki pants and khaki shirt through the hatch. Lanes gave me my boots, and my boots had my inmate number on the bottom of the heel. It read *73223*. I began to dress into my clothing and my boots. It usually took me about five minutes to fully dress myself. Lanes put me in full body chains, which took another five minutes. After that I was all set to go. I was taken through the large gate and passed the control unit doors. Then I was taken to the elevator and up the elevator. From there I was led through the hallway. The hallway was long, and I had to pass all the units to get to the visiting. Then I had to climb the stairs, which had about thirty steps. From the steps I was in the strip out station. The strip out station was never fun because I had to get naked each time I was in front of the officers. The strip out station was small and had a mirror against the back wall. The mirror was large, and it was in the shape of a square. There was also a window that peered out towards the big yard, and the window had blinds on it.

"Strip Bower," Floos said.

Floos was the visiting officer in charge. Floos had a widow's peak and a long nose. He was white and had blue eyes.

"So Bower, who is here to see you today?" he asked me while I was stripping naked.

"Your mommy?" he said.

He began to laugh at me, and his laugh was very annoying, and it added to his ugly personality.

"Bend over, Bower," Floos said.

Floos was a real piece of work, and he could be really mean or really messed up at times. There was no being nice with this guy. He was holding the chain restraints, swinging them back and forth. He began to swing the chains my direction.

"Oops," Floos said.

"Did I almost hit you in the sack, Bower? Maybe next time I will hit you right in your balls," he said.

"I would tell on you," I said.

"Who would believe you? You're just a piece of shit

inmate," Floos said.

I could tell Floos was trying to make me upset right before my visit with my mom.

"I would tell my mom," I said.

"Ya, and what's mommy gonna do?"

"My mom would report it," I said.

"Do you hear yourself right now?"

Floos was in my face while talking. He thought it was funny, and I knew it was wrong. Afterwards I would go into my visit with my mom lost for words. I wouldn't know what to say. In some visits I wouldn't even talk for minutes, and my mom would just sit there looking at me with hurt and concern. My mom knew bad things were happening, but there was very little that she could do about it. I would leave my visit hugging my mother in chains. I was never able to get used to the hugs. I couldn't give my mother a full hug at all. I would tell my mother that I loved her and goodbye. From there we parted ways, and I often watched my mom leave in worry. I would be escorted back to the strip out room by Floos and Wallace. They were both the male visiting officers. Floos would stand over me as I would be stripping, and he would begin talking shit.

"So what did you and your mommy talk about?"

"Nothing," I said.

"You're damn right you talked about nothing," Wallace said.

Then Wallace cracked a smile as if he were joking. It wasn't a joke to me though. Wallace was white and had a shaved head, and his eyes were blue. He had a short nose and he wasn't very tall.

"Bower, can you do push ups with your full body chains on?" Floos was asking.

"No," I said.

"Ya, can you?" Wallace said.

"I don't know," I said.

I was unsure if I could, but I also didn't care.

"Come on, do a push up," Floos said.

He was taunting me now.

"Come on, I will even help you to the floor," he said.

He grabbed my arm, and I began to follow his lead.

"That's right, get down there," he said. "Face down all the way."

I eventually made it to the floor, and Floos stood over me, and he placed his genitals over my head and started doing a humping motion. I couldn't get up on my own because of the chain restraints.

"How do you like that, Bower? Your head is getting fucked," Floos said.

"Ya, you're a good bitch, Bower," Wallace said.

Wallace was standing in front of Floos while my forehead was hitting the carpet.

"Get off me," I said.

"No, you will stay down there," Floos said.

"Get off me," I repeated.

I was in a very uncomfortable position.

"Okay, let him up," Wallace said.

They both helped me up off of the ground and acted like they did nothing wrong.

"Bower, get the fuck out of my sight," Floos said.

I went back to my cell feeling emotional pain. I was hurt, and there was nothing that I could do about it. Floos was right—I was just a piece of shit inmate. Who would ever believe me? The worst part is that's how it would be each and every visit. I was abused, and if I said anything I was a snitch. It seemed that no one really cared other than my mother. Floos seemed to have no regard of emotion to me as a human being. Wallace turned a blind eye each time, and sometimes Wallace would help Floos. Like the time I went up to see my mother and Floos wanted to have fun with me. He wanted to break me before I went into my visit. Floos and Wallace grabbed both of my arms. Then they turned me towards the mirror. They both walked me up to the mirror and began telling me to kiss it.

"Kiss the mirror, Bower," Floos said.

"No," I said.

"Shut up and stop talking," he said.

"Now kiss the fucking mirror," Floos said.

"Kiss it," Wallace said.

I knew if I didn't do what they wanted, I would regret it later. At the same time, I didn't want to give them satisfaction for what they were doing. So I did as they directed me to, and I kissed the mirror.

"Mush!"

"Ya," Wallace said.

"We got Bower to kiss the fucking mirror."

"Kiss the mirror," Floos mocked.

"That was a good one," Wallace said.

I went into the visit with my mother, and all I could do was cry. I cried for two minutes telling my mother what just happened. She was angry, and I could see in her eyes that she wanted justice. However, there was very little my mother could do. I was broken by all the pain and suffering that I had endured. The past four years hadn't really been the greatest for me, and I just wanted it to be over. I counted down the days that I had left to serve while I was in my cell.

"Seven hundred and forty-nine days," I said.

That's a long ways away, I thought. By now I was doing much better, and I realized that I had to ignore the other inmates around me if I ever wanted to leave the control unit. I had my bunk back and my mattress back too. Even my clothing I had back. I had all my canteen privileges so I could purchase my store products. I also had my pens with my paper and my envelopes. I was moving up in the world of the control unit. I was close to getting out of cell sixteen, and I'd been in this cell for nearly nine months. I continued to go to visiting each time that I had a visitor. One time I was on the phone with a friend named Ashley Phinox. I knew her from the community, and she wanted to see me. So she arranged a visit for Wednesday. So that following Wednesday I told the sergeant that I had a visitor coming to see me. I told him in the morning hours, and I thought nothing of it. Well visiting time arrived, and I had no call for my visit. So I waited patiently for the sergeant to come and chain me up for my visit. Still no one showed to escort me, and I knew my visitor was here because lunch just finished. I began to wonder if she even came. A few hours went by and the sergeant finally came out with an escort to chain me up. I was given my khakis and my boots, and I was sent to visiting. When I arrived to visiting it took another five minutes to strip out. By that time my visitor was preparing to leave. Ashley had brown hair and brown eyes, and her nose was short. She was a very attractive women. She had

302

light tan skin, and she wasn't very tall.

"What took you so long?"

"I don't know," I said.

"Well, I have to leave soon, Austin. Can I get you anything?"

"Ya, can I please have a soda?"

"Sure," she said.

Ashley stayed for five minutes, and in those five minutes she bought me a candy bar and a soda pop. Then soon after she had to leave. I told Ashley that I didn't know why it took so long, but I knew why. I knew why all too well. It was that piece of shit sergeant, and I was foolish to think telling him about my visit was okay. Well it wasn't, and it taught me that these fuckers were my number one enemy. They hated me so much that they made me wait two hours while my visitor sat here waiting for me. My visitor wasn't happy at all, and who could blame her? It wasn't her fault; she didn't know, but I should've known. Yet I told that worthless coward sensitive information that I should not have. Nevertheless, I learned from it, and what I learned is you can't trust someone who chains you up every day. Once a snake always a snake, and that's why other inmates say keep your grass cut low. They say that with all seriousness, so you are more careful with what you are doing and who you're doing it around.

303

Another thing about visiting is my mother would visit me on a regular basis. I was blessed to have a mother who would come to see me all the time. She would bring me money for the vending machines and spend countless quarters on me. My mother spent over two thousand dollars on me during my stay at the Lincoln Correctional Center. She would buy me soda and chips, candy bars and honey buns. My mom showed me love through it all, and I could never thank her enough for it. She would talk to me about God and how Jesus needs to be the center of my life. I listened to my mother, and I had faith in what she would preach. Also that one day justice would be swift for all the things these prison officials did to me. That one day was coming, and through it all God would see me make it out of this evil prison system.

The visiting staff wouldn't allow me to bring a Bible in for my mother, and they wouldn't allow her to bring a Bible in for me. There was a separate system for that, and it was called clergy visiting. Only a pastor could bring in a Bible to study the word of God with an inmate, which was really hard because there were limits on who you could have as a clergy visitor. Those limits would often conflict with my faith. So most often I would go without a clergy pastor, and I would read the word of God in my cell. My days of visiting were tough, and it was a challenge to have my mom see me chained up everytime I came through those doors. I hated it so much, and I knew if I didn't get out of segregation sooner rather than later, I would soon hate myself. My brother was another advocate that I had. He would visit me and buy me soda. He bought me candy as well while I sat with him. He would get the dominos out from the activity closet. The activity closet was there for times such as these. My brother would play me in dominos, and I would win most of the time.

"J.R.," I said.

"What's up, bro?"

"Can you start sending me money?"

"How much money?"

"Fifty dollars a month," I said.

"Ya, I can do that. What do you need it for?"

"Hygiene supplies and food," I said. "I also need it for phone time and envelopes."

"Okay," he said.

Ever since then I would receive fifty dollars a month from my brother in the mail. It was a blessing really. I had no other way of making money. I wasn't given a job in segregation, and I sat there to waste away. My brother really looked out for me too. It was money that I needed, and money I wouldn't of had without him. I had needs, and my brother provided during times that were tight for him. I can't ever thank him enough for that. He was loyal to me, and that made our bond much stronger with one another. I was thankful for my mother and my brother. Occasionally my little sister would visit me as well, and she made things pleasant. Her innocence in such a dark place helped me survive the evil things about prison. After the visit was the hardest part because I had to decompress from leaving my family and watching them walk away. Knowing that I had to stay and they didn't made things hard for me. Moreover, them leaving and I couldn't leave with them. I would never want them to stay in a place like this. My family helped me by supporting me during my sentence in prison. By them visiting me showed me that they loved me, and I needed that in such a dark place. I will always be thankful for the times they sacrificed to come see me in this shit hole. I can understand that it wasn't an easy place to visit a loved one.

Chapter 26 Dr. Pretzel

An Estimated 40,168 individuals in Nebraska have serious mental illness, and are below 200% of the poverty level.

I progressed where I was located by maintaining on the base line system that was designed to modify behavior. It was a system that in all honesty didn't work for the most part. No one cared if they received a check mark or not. At least for the most part other inmates thought it was horse shit. I did too, but if I ever wanted to get out of this cell, I had to follow their rules by their system. As the old saying goes, their house their rules. I was only a guest in their house, and I didn't want to stay as a guest for long. I wanted out of this hellish environment, and I wanted out as soon as possible. I had no check marks for over two months on my base line, and that was a good feeling to have.

"Bower, get ready," Dickerson said.

Dickerson was new to the facility, and I could smell the fear on him.

"For what?"

"You have a meeting with mental health," he said.

"Who in mental health?"

"I think his name is Dr. Pretzel," he said.

"Man, I have to see him again?"

"I don't make the rules," Dickerson said. "You can refuse if you want."

I wasn't too thrilled to have this meeting, and I had seen Pretzel before. I would speak of my autism, and Pretzel didn't seem interested. My mother even sent him documentation in regards to my autism. Yet he found a loophole not to provide treatment. Dickerson was standing at the gate while he was talking to me.

"Anyways, get ready," Dickerson said.

Dickerson was fat and large with a country boy accent. Dickerson was real country, and he knew it too. He came from the middle of Nebraska, a real breadwinner. He was new here, and tried to play it off like he wasn't scared. However, I could smell the fear all over him. Dickerson placed me in full body restraints and escorted me to the elevator.

"So, what are you going to talk about in there?"

"I don't know," I said.

"Are you gonna bitch about how bad this place is?"

"You know, that's not a bad idea," I said. "But no, I plan to talk about my diagnosis."

"Why?"

"Because they gave me a false diagnosis," I said.

308

"What are they saying you have?"

"Borderline personality disorder," I said.

"And what do you have?"

"Autism."

Dickerson looked me over for a few seconds.

"You don't look autistic," he said.

"Are you a doctor?"

"Still you don't seem autistic," he said.

"Again are you a doctor?"

"No, I'm not," he said.

The elevator came to a stop, and Dickerson began to lead the way.

"Well, since you're not a doctor," I said, "how would you know what another human being would or would not have? You never went to school for it."

We were both walking as I was talking to Dickerson. The ankle chains were making noise on the tile floors.

"Ya, well I have a girlfriend, and her kid has autism," he said.

"How do you know if it's autism?"

"I don't know," he said. "But that's what my girlfriend told me."

"My point," I said.

"Okay, let's leave it alone, Bower."

"You brought it up," I said.

"Ya, okay," he said.

Dickerson led me through the hallwall, nearing the mental health office.

I was able to hear the radio on Dickerson's shoulder. There were small beeps and various noises. Once we approached the door, Dickerson unlocked it. From there he led me in, and he instructed me to take a seat. There were a row of chairs in the mental health office, and I sat in the chair that was in the corner. A receptionist was seated at her desk answering phone calls and writing things down on her notepad. She had puffy hair, and she was tall with beady eyes. She had white skin and pink fingernail polish.

"Hello, Austin," she said.

"Hello, Bethany," I said.

"How are you doing?"

"I'm okay," I said.

I lied, I was far from okay.

"Austin, did you know I used to work with your father, Jeff?"

"Really?"

"Isn't that cool?"

310

"Yes, that's cool," I said.

My escort had a disgusted look on his face.

"Out of all the times I've seen you, I never had the chance to tell you," she said.

"Well, I know now," I said.

"Yes, you do. Your father was a great man."

"Thank you," I said.

"It's too bad he died at such a young age," she said.

"I know."

"He was only forty-two," she said.

"I know."

The mental health office was flowing with traffic. Mental health counselors were coming and going. Filing paperwork and printing copies off of the computer scanner. There was a printer in the main office to the lobby. I could see two doors that led to two different conference rooms. One of the conference rooms was for morning meetings. There was a hallway that led to the back of the mental health office. Towards the back of the hallway were six different units. Within those units were offices, and each office had a designated doctor or counselor.

"Mr. Bower," Pretzel said.

Dr. Pretzel was thin like a pretzel, so his name fit his personality well. He was bony and wore glasses. He had brown eyes and gray hair.

"Hello, Dr. Pretzel," I said.

"Hello, Mr. Bower."

"Here, come on back," he said.

"I have a question for you, Dr. Pretzel," I said.

"Okay shoot."

I took a seat in his office, and he managed to take a seat in his leather chair. Dickerson waited outside of the room. Dr. Pretzel's room was well organized with books and a nice looking computer. He also had a filing cabinet that leaned against his back wall.

"Why is my counselor continuing to tell me that I don't have autism?"

"Because you don't," he said.

"Come on, Dr. Pretzel, my mother gave you documentation on my autism," I said.

"Well, she gave us documentation," he said, "but not in the regards to autism. You see, when you were a child, you had signs of borderline personality disorder."

"I don't have borderline personality disorder," I said.

"Well the documentation says differently," he said.

"So, even know the DSMs speak about how children should not be diagnosed with personality disorders," I said.

312

"Because it is frowned upon," he said.

"Then why do you feel the need to believe your reason?"

"My diagnosis for you will stay the same," he said.

"So what are my chances of returning to the mental health unit?"

"You don't have one," he said. "Your disorder is not a severe diagnosis."

"So I have no chance of returning to Delta unit?"

"No," he said. "Unfortunately you don't."

"Was it your idea to place me on full beds?"

"What?"

"On five point for over three weeks?"

"I don't know what you are talking about," he said.

"Sure you do," I said.

"You mean in the infirmary? On five point?"

"Yes," I said.

"Wow, they kept you on five-point for over three weeks?"

"Yes, for over three weeks," I said. "But something tells me you knew about it."

"No, I didn't," he said.

"Then who was it?"

"I'm not sure," he said. "Do you have any more questions?"

"No."

"Okay, I want to ask you something, Mr. Bower. So why are you not taking your meds?"

"Because I am angry," I said.

"So staying off of your medication will help?"

"No," I said.

"Mr. Bower, I want to start you on a new pill," he said.

"Okay, what is it called?"

"It's called Stellizen," he said.

"Okay, whats it for?"

"It's for mood disorder," he said.

"Why do you want me on that?"

"Because I believe it will help you. So I will write you a prescription for this week. You should start receiving the new medication in about a day or two."

"Okay," I said.

"Okay, Mr. Bower, I think we are all done here," he said.

Dr. Pretzel stood up and opened the door, and he led me out to my escort.

"All done?"

"Yes," I said.

"I was asking the doctor," Dickerson said.

"Oh," I said.

"Yes, we are done," Pretzel said.

"Great, take care, Doc," Dickerson said.

I was led back to my cell the same way we came. Nothing was said between me and Dickerson on the way back. Our feelings about each other were mutual. I thought he was a piece of shit, and he thought I was a piece of shit. I was taken back to my cell, which I hated returning to. It was small and cold. I was still in cell sixteen, and I hated it so much, but what could I do about it. Time was not on my watch; it was on their watch. All I could do was accept it for what it was, and that is what I did. If I tried to fight it, it would cost me. I already lost two years of good time, and I was trying to earn those two years back. My initial discharge date had already come to pass, and I was going nowhere until I earned my good time back.

Chapter 27 The Oath

The (CDC) reported those with (ASD) Autism Spectrum Disorder are 6.2 percent times greater in medical costs per year. And those with (ASD) including adults with (ASD) Spend $6,200 more dollars on medical bills each year. Compared to those who do not have (ASD).

I was moved from cell sixteen to cell nine, and I didn't know what took the administration so long to move me. I was moved, and that's all that mattered. I was happy to be where I was. I mean I wasn't happy in the sense of freedom happy; rather, I was happy in the sense I wouldn't be watched by the camera any more happy. That camera made me unhappy, and it's not like I was on camera for a movie or anything. No, I was watched to be reminded that I was scum, and they could watch me whenever they wanted to. That camera made me feel so uncomfortable and less human. They watched me while I was naked and while I had nothing to my name. It was evident that they hated me, and I could feel the hatred from their hearts directed towards me. It pierced my heart, and I could feel their swords piercing me. I was unsure of how long I would stay in this cell, but I was also unsure about life in general. I just didn't know what direction to go in. I felt abandoned by my God, and I felt like he wasn't near. Nevertheless, I still prayed to him over and over again. I believed that he heard my cries, and I believed he saw my tears. I believed he could feel my heartbeat, and I believed he loved me. I was at the point in my life that I had to make a decision of who my friends were going to be. I believe I made a decision right where I was. I sat at my desk, and I told my heavenly father words that I will never forget.

"No more," I prayed.

I was praying, and my head was on the desk as I sat at my desk.

"No more weed and no more drugs," I prayed. "No more. God, I give you an oath. I will do right, God, and I will discharge successfully. I will make it out. I won't hang around people like Hawkboy ever again. I give you my word, God. I will stay away from all of that, all of that that brought me here. I mean it, God."

I was crying as tears were falling down my face. I had been in prison for three years, and I longed to discharge, and I knew what that meant. I knew what I had to do to make it out. I knew that life was more precious than what these guards made life out to be. So I ignored all the inmates who would provoke me. I knew better than to engage with them in an argument. I had no friends here, and I knew it too. I knew that I needed to ignore them to make it up to C unit. So I gave an oath to God that I would strive to discharge, and that meant no more threats and no more yelling. That meant I would just lay down. I would lay my time down on my mattress. I realized I couldn't win any other way. I realized that this was the only way I could do it. It was the only way that I could fight back. It was my secret weapon, and it was a tool that I could use to help me in any situation. I used my mattress as a scapegoat. Whenever they yelled at me, I laid down on my mattress. I knew that it was the only honest way to avoid all of the chaos that I had been dealing with. I didn't ever want to go back to the metal table again.

I was tired of the mental health staff telling me that I didn't have autism. I was sick and tired of Dr. Pretzel and his lies. He knew he was a liar too. I was tired of all the verbal abuse I had to deal with, and I was tired of being told what to do all the time. I was around evil every day, and it wasn't getting any better. I was stuck around inmates who would be here for the rest of their lives. I was stuck around people that I didn't claim. I knew that I didn't claim these people because I was better than them. I was at the wrong place at the wrong time with the wrong person. That in itself cost me my life for a few years if not more. My felony would make things harder for me to find a job, even if I was qualified to do the work. Nevertheless, I needed out, and I knew this would be a long fight. So I made an oath to God, in hopes that God would have my back in the process.

Chapter 28 Parole

The Autism Society estimates that 60% of annual costs of autism are from the needs of adults on the spectrum, in particular for residential care across the adult lifespan.

"Bower, do you want to see the parole board?"

I thought about the idea for a moment before I replied. "Yes," I said.

"Okay, get ready," Lue said.

Lue was fat and out of shape. I learned that whenever a guard said 'get ready' what they really meant was hurry up and wait. So I did nothing, and I just sat at my desk until they were ready for me. I waited about twenty minutes, and then Lue brought me my khaki pants and my khaki shirt along with my boots. I began to dress, and I dressed slowly. I figured I wouldn't get parole, but hey I had the same amount of chances as the next guy. I finished getting dressed, and then Lue ran my cell door. Lue was slow with his hands as he began placing the chain restraints on me.

"Do you think you will get parole, Bower?"

I looked Lue over.

"I don't know, only time will tell," I said.

"Yes, it will," he said.

After I was chained up and ready, Lue escorted me to the elevator and through the control unit door.

"So if you don't get parole, how will you react?"

"I don't know," I said. "That's a very odd question."

"Just something to think about," he said. "Most people in the control unit get turned down."

"Really?"

"Yes," he said.

"Well, wish me luck then," I said.

"You'll need all the luck that you can get," he said.

I continued walking down the hallway, and I didn't feel like talking anymore. I figured I would walk in silence the rest of the way there. I reached the turning doors to the next hallway, and from there my escort walked me to the library. The parole board hearing was being held in the back of the library. There was a general population inmate doing the preparation for the parole board intake. He was black with brown hair and brown eyes. He had a tattoo of a blood symbol on his right arm. Lue directed me to follow him into the library. Lue unlocked the library door. Then Lue walked me into the room with the black inmate. Lue had me take a seat in the small room, and Lue shut the door behind him. Lue stationed himself near the front entrance of the library. The black inmate was holding a brown clipboard and shuffling papers.

"Name?"

"Bower," I said.

"Number?"

"73223," I said.

"Wait here until the board calls you back," he said.

I saw three board members seated in the library. One member was a tall black male, and the other two members were both white females. All three of them had computers in front of them. The black man signaled to Lue with his hand, and Lue went closer to the blackboard member. Lue leaned over to communicate with the tall black board member. Then Lue walked my direction, and he opened the door to the room that I was in.

"Come take a seat, Bower," Lue said.

I walked out towards the board members, and I took a seat right in front of them.

"State your name and number for the record," the black board member said.

There was a microphone in front of me, and the black board member made eye contact with me.

"Austin Bower," I said.

"Your number?"

321

"73223," I said.

"Mr. Bower, you are in the control unit," he said.

"Yes," I said.

"You had six misconduct reports in the past three months," he said.

"Yes," I said.

"You also haven't finished the violent offenders program," he said.

"No, I haven't."

"Well, stay misconduct report free for one year," he said, "and finish the violent offenders program."

"Then what?"

"Then we will talk about parole," he said. "Your next parole hearing will be scheduled for next year. You may be dismissed, Mr. Bower."

I had mixed emotions about what just happened, and I began to wonder why I even came. I had my head down the entire time I walked back to my cell. I was escorted and placed back into cell nine. I hated what just happened, and I couldn't get over it, but I had an oath to keep to God. I was obligated to keep this oath too. So I stuck it out, and I walked with my head held high. I was escorted back to my cell by Lue, and he didn't say a word during my return.

Chapter 29 The Move

"Bower, pack your shit. We're moving you up to C unit," Copley said. He opened my hatch, and he handed me a plastic bag. I began to pack my soap and shampoo and my radio. I packed my books and my legal pad. I also packed my envelopes and my pens. I was ready to go after two long years of being trapped in the control unit. I was in cell sixteen for one year, and it was horrific. I hated every second of it. I was in cell nine before that for two months, and after cell sixteen, I was in cell nine for ten months. I was headed back to C unit where I first started, and I was hoping for it to be a positive transition. My escort came down to chain me up in full body chains, and then I was led to the elevator. My escort carried all of my belongings for me. He was dark skinned, and he had brown eyes with brown hair, and he was tall. He was about six foot four in height. After the elevator, he led me through the elevator doors and into the hallway after he received clearance.

"Hogs to Charlie," he said. "I have one at your door."

It took the charlie unit staff about five minutes to

finally get to the unit door. Once they did I was let in by a short caseworker named Brutis. I had prior experience with him in the past.

"Come on in, Bower," Brutis said.

He seemed to have a wit about him.

"You will be housed in upper one," he said.

I was led up a flight of stairs by both my escort and Brutis. Hogs unchained me at the cell door. Brutis took my property and put it aside.

"I will need to search your items, Bower, before I return them to you," he said.

"Why?"

"It's policy," he said.

"Okay."

Brutis shut the door and removed the cuffs from my hands through the hatch.

"Get comfortable, Bower," Brutis said.

I went to the back of my cell, and I laid on my mattress. I laid there until dinnertime, and a set of new caseworkers were on the unit to take over. The caseworkers were Grans and Bonus. They were passing out mail to all the inmates, and I received a three hundred dollar money order from my mom in the mail.

'*Happy Birthday,*' the letter read.

There was a note inside the letter that wished me the best.

"Is it August already?"

I knew what to do with the money, and that was buy a television with it.

The very next day I received a money order and a birthday card from my brother, Justin.

'*Happy Birthday,*' the letter read.

"Is it your birthday, do bear bears shit in woods?"

There was a picture of a bear on the front of the card. The bear was taking a dump in the woods. I received fifty dollars from my brother for the things I needed while living in segregation, such as soap, shampoo, toothpaste, and a new toothbrush. I also bought some food items as well. The food that I bought was often candy or chocolate. The food was never anything healthy. There were soups and bags of chips, which I bought from time to time. I learned to lay my time down and to relax during hardships and negative situations. There were caseworkers that would try to make me angry, but I had a goal. That goal was to discharge back to the streets. I had a little over a year left before I could discharge. I still had good time to earn back, which I was doing by staying out of trouble and not making any verbal threats to anyone. I called my mother on the telephone, and she picked up right away.

"Hey Mom," I said.

"Did you get the money?"

"Ya, I got the money, Mom," I said.

"Are you going to buy a television?"

"Ya, I am," I said.

"Make sure you do," she said.

"Okay, Mom I will. I love you, Mom," I said.

"I love you too, honey," she said.

"So how is Justin doing?"

"He's good," she said. "Did you get his money?"

"Ya, I got it."

"Good."

"Okay Mom, I will talk with you soon," I said.

"Okay, honey, I love you."

"I love you too, Mom. Okay, have a good night."

"You too," she said.

After that I hung up and I set the phone on the hatch to my cell door. I had a radio that I listened to, and I listened to the Christian radio news. I would get updates about what was happening in the Middle East. I took a direct order form, and I purchased my television. I bought a remote control separately. The downfall was I had to wait eight weeks to receive my television. Nevertheless, I had time to kill, so I figured eight weeks wasn't hardly a wait at all, considering how much time I had already done in prison. This was nothing that I couldn't handle. I put my order in, and that was that.

For the next eight weeks I went to yard and had my visits with my family. I would write poetry and stories on my notepad. My poems were in regards to my dreams and my ambitions that I had in life. I would lay on my mattress and think of fun memories. I also had bad memories too. I would think about my father sometimes and what he went through. He received his degree in psychology while being an on side alcoholic. Nevertheless, he achieved it, and for that I looked up to my father. I often thought of memories of how abusive he was to me. He smoked cigarettes, and the smoking took his life. I looked back at those days in my mind when I was at his funeral. I often wondered what it would be like if he was still around. That is a question that only God could answer, I suppose.

My days often drug out into the nighttime hours, so sometimes during the day I would sleep. At night it was so quiet that I enjoyed the peace. So I would stay up late just to write a song or a poem. I loved to write, and I even often thought about being published some day. I dreamed about how my book would be on the shelves throughout America and that I would have respect from those such as Steven King and

James Patterson. I even enjoyed books from Walter Dean Myers and his book slam. I read often, and it was a good habit to get myself into. So that's what I did, and I figured if someday I wanted to be published, what better thing to do than read. I can't count the books that I have read, especially ones that I have enjoyed. My favorites would have to be John Sanford and David Schickler. I enjoyed Schickler's book *Kissing in Manhattan*. I've even enjoyed a few Dean Koontz' books, one of which is *Odd Thomas*. I love books that I can't put down. It's the thrill of reading, and knowledge is just such a powerful thing. Reading most definitely gives you knowledge. So on rainy days that I had in prison I would read. I have also read books from C.S. Lewis and the *Screw Tape Letters*. I have even read C.S. Lewis' *Mere Christianity*, and *The Great Divorce*. All three of those books I enjoyed reading. Books like that really stick with you too. They give you a sense of what it's like to finish something. The way they wrote to their audiences and how they connected with us is mesmerizing. So during my time of waiting I would divert my attention to a good book.

I waited the eight week period out patiently, and sure enough my Hiteker television came in the mail, and I was all set for business.

"Bower," Shelly said.

Shelly was the canteen lady, and I and all the inmates called her canteen.

"Your television is here," she said.

"Great," I said.

"I will need you to sign for the order," she said.

"Okay."

She opened the hatch and handed me my remote control and had me sign for my television. The hatch was too small for the television to fit through, so caseworker Bonus had to give me my television by unlocking my cell door.

"Stand back in your cell," Bonus said.

Bonus was working the unit tonight, and I got along with him okay.

"Now turn around and face the wall," he said.

I did as he instructed, and the next thing I knew I had a television. I had a chair in my room, and I hooked up my television to my coaxial cables. I had a wall jack in my cell for cable use. There was a wall jack inside every cell. However, there were no wall jacks in the cells of the control unit. After I hooked my television up, I set my television on my chair, and I laid down on my mattress. I received thirteen channels through the cable jack, five of which were local channels. My television helped me pass time by, and I treated my television right. I wouldn't tug on it, and I also wouldn't drag it. I was very careful with my television because it was important to me. It was my key to survival, and books only lasted so long until they became tiresome. Reading requires exercise because when you read, you're working your mind. That's why most people read before they go to bed, because it's a healthy way to fall asleep. My days were still slow, but having a television made things much easier on me. The months seemed to fly by after receiving my television. Matter of fact, I couldn't believe how fast time began to go by. 'Thanks Mom, you are appreciated,' I would often lip to myself while watching a film.

Having a television made a serious move in how well I did with ignoring other inmates. There was still one inmate who caused hell for everybody. He would wake everyone up in the middle of the night. He was a small black man, and his name was Edda Albums. Edda was a sex offender, and he raped his nine-year-old nephew in a public bathroom in Omaha, Nebraska. The only reason why he could walk the yard was because of his brother. He was the brother of a shot caller for the Crips. His brother ran eighty two inmates of the Lincoln Correctional Center. His brother didn't care that he was a sex offender, but others did. This motherfucker would pound on his door at three in the morning just to have his blood sugar checked. The crazy thing was he didn't even have diabetes. He woke everyone up, but no one else said anything. The other inmates feared his brother; however, I didn't fear him at all. Plus I knew that I wasn't going back to Delta unit. Also the administration placed me on involuntary protective custody. So I was screwed in that regard, but I knew it would never come back to harm me. So at times when he pissed me off I would provoke him because I knew that I could. He woke me up, so I gave him a piece of my mind. I would do to him what other inmates did to me. It was a sense of survival in a way, and I needed to get some frustration out. Plus it's not like he was special in any regard; I mean, come on, he raped his nephew. That is the lowest form of human life. I believe in values, and I even have morals. However, if you woke me up at three in the morning, and I knew you were a sex offender, I would talk trash to you until sun up. I would run my mouth until you wanted to fight me. Also I wanted peace and quiet. I didn't want to hear some rapist run his mouth about needing his blood sugar checked, especially at three in the morning. I couldn't believe this guy could walk the yard. In some states if inmates knew you were a sex offender, you had to go straight to protective custody. Unfortunately, Nebraska isn't one of those states, and it probably never will be.

Chapter 30 A-Unit

The signs of autism in adults are as followed: 1 significant problems developing nonverbal communication skills which include eye contact, facial expressions, and body posture.

"Mr. Bower," Duke said.

"May I have a word with you?"
"Sure," I said.

He was holding a set of papers in his hands. He also had a pen clipped to his button shirt. His shirt was a three piece button shirt, such as a polo. His slacks were brown, and I noticed how they looked ironed. He walked with a cane everywhere he went. Rumor has it Duke was jumped by three black inmates. He was fairly new at the time, and the inmates didn't like him. I was told this was back in the early nineteen nineties.

"Mr. Bower, you are doing exceptionally well," he said. "But we want to see how well you do with others. So we want you to go to protective custody. From there we can see about sending you back to delta unit. So are you willing to go?"

"Yes," I said.

I was standing at my cell door.

"Then I will need you to sign this form for me, and we can get you moved today," he said.

Duke slide the form through the door, and I signed it on my desk. Then I slid the form back to Duke. Duke was headed back to his office to finalize the order. I waited a few hours in my cell by laying on my mattress. Then I soon decided to stand near my cell door. I noticed a guard standing at the bottom of the steps, and he was looking at me. His name was Judges, and he was tall. He had short hair and green eyes.

"Bower, are you ready to go?"

I looked his direction, and I said nothing to him at all. Judges held a plastic bag in his hand, and he soon came up to my cell. He unlocked my hatch, and he then handed me the plastic bag.

"Here, pack your things," he said.

I packed all of my belongings, and then he opened my cell door. I was out of my cell with no cuffs and no chain restraints after having to wear cuffs and chain restraints for over two years. This was a big change for me, and I didn't like it. I had my television in one hand and my belongings in the other.

"Let's get you to A-unit," he said.

Judges walked me out of my cell, and he escorted me to A-unit. We took the long way through turnkey, and he led me through two large doors. Once we arrived to A-unit, Judges radioed for the caseworker.

"Judges to A-unit," he said. "I have one at your spin."

The case worker came walking towards the spin door, and he unlocked the door quickly.

The caseworker was older and had aging white hair. His name was King, and he was fairly tall. If I had to guess, he was probably six foot three.

"You must be Bower," he said. "I got it from here, Judges," King said.

Judges left while shutting the door behind him.

"I'm caseworker King. I will take you to your cell. You will be housed with inmate Parks. He doesn't cause trouble for anyone," King said.

King led me to my cell. We walked past the main office and down a flight of stairs. Parks was white, and he was young. I could see Parks through the cell window. King opened the cell door, and I entered the cell that Parks was in. King shut the door behind me and walked away. I saw a few centerfolds on Parks' desk, and he had a flat screen television. I laid my plastic bag on the floor, and I placed my television on top of a small dresser. I saw two blue chairs, and I took a seat in the chair closest to the toilet.

"Hey man, what's good?"

334

"You know, living the dream," he said.

"How much time are you doing?"

"I'm doing sixty years," he said.

"No shit," I said.

"No shit's right. Well you have the top bunk, and I have the bottom bunk."

I looked at the top bunk, and I thought this thing was going to be a bitch to climb. I hated where I was at from the moment I walked in. I couldn't believe this, and I thought how I wish I would have stayed in the hole. I was so used to it, and it became normal to me. I hated being with another person, and I guess that's because I was in the hole for so long. I had to get the fuck out of there, I thought. This wasn't what I wanted, and it wasn't what I wanted to do. I had to get the fuck out of there. Fuck this, I thought, I don't want to be here. I wanted my own cell, and I wanted to be alone.

"Caseworker," I said.

I began pounding on the cell door, and the door made loud thud noises.

"Caseworker please let me out of here," I said.

"Hey caseworker!"

"Who is that?"

"It's me, Bower," I said.

"What do you want, Bower?"

"I want to be let out, please."

"Well, Bower, I can't let you out," he said.

"I want to go back to the hole."

"Why?"

"Because I can't stand this place," I said.

"I can't send you back without a reason," he said.

"I fear for my safety."

I was lying to him, and I knew it too.

"Bower, what's wrong?"

"Everything," I said.

"Okay, I will have you escorted."

King walked away and headed up the stairs.

"Man, are you okay?" Parks asked me while he was seated on his bunk.

"No, not really," I said.

"Well, it was nice knowing you," Parks said.

I waited about twenty minutes until my escort showed up, and I had all my belongings packed. My escort was black, and he had tattoos on his forearms. My escort unlocked the cell door.

"Turn around," he said. "I need to put these cuffs on you."

"Okay," I said.

I was placed in the handcuffs and escorted back to the hole.

Chapter 31 The Hole

The sign of autism in adults are as followed: 2 The inability, and failure to establish friendship with other adults who are the same age.

I was sent back to the hole in hopes that I would have the same cell that I had before. I wasn't given the same cell though, and that's what really drove me mad. I should have known better though. I was housed in the lower level of C-unit. I was escorted by Officer Lock, and I was still in handcuffs. Lock was black, and he had tiger tattoos on his forearms. I wasn't given the same cell, however I was on the same unit. It seemed to only get worse one day at a time. I should have never left segregation from the beginning, I thought. My hope was to earn my good time back so I could discharge. There was still light at the end of the tunnel. I was placed into a cell that smelled of sewer water, and the water was all over the cell floor. The water was black, and it came from the sprinkler head in the cell. It was popped one hour before I moved in, and the cell toilet was flooded too. My mattress was soaked in sewer water, and I was given new bed sheets, but that didn't make a difference. The water seeped through the bed sheets, and I could feel the water soaking my white shirt. I

338

had no inkling of what I had to do. The smell was dreadful, and it was disgusting in many ways. I had no choice but to get the attention of the correctional staff.

"Hey caseworker," I said. "Can any one hear me? I need some help!"

I continued to try to get the attention of the correctional staff. However, they continued to ignore me.

"I need a new mattress," I said.

I continued yelling, and I was ignored for over ten minutes.

"What the hell do you want?"

The caseworker looked angry. He wore glasses, and he had a beard.

He wasn't very tall at all, and he walked away quickly to avoid me.

"Hey caseworker," I said.

I began to pound on the cell door.

"What do you want?"

"I need a new mattress," I said.

"What's wrong with the one you have?"

"It has sewer water in it," I said.

"Well suck it up," he said.

After his statement he walked away.

"Hey come back," I said. "Please!"

Nothing for the next two hours, and I didn't hear as little as a pen drop.

"Hey, I need a new mattress," I said.

I kept this up for the next thirty minutes, yelling for a new mattress. I was ignored the entire night, and no one cared that I had to sleep on a sewer infested mattress. By the time I knew it, the lights went out, and no one was going to help me. I was forced to sleep on this filthy mattress. So I made do, and I laid down. The entire night I was tossing and turning, and somehow the sewer water got into my mouth. It was very disgusting, and I rose off the mattress to brush my teeth.

"Gross," I said.

The very next day I called my mother, and I told her what was happening. She became frantic, and she revealed worry in her voice.

"Okay, are they going to get you a new mattress?"

"I don't know," I said.

"What do you mean you don't know?"

"Like I said, I don't know. I've been asking for over two days,

and they still haven't done anything about it," I said.

"Okay," she said.

She took a deep breath.

"I will see what I can do."

I didn't say anything at all.

"Are you okay, Austin?"

I sat there saying nothing, and then I began to cry.

"Mom, I want you to save me," I said. "Please come in here and save me."

I was sobbing out tears.

"Honey, don't cry. I will do my best," she said.

"You have one minute remaining," the phone said.

"I love you, Austin."

"I love you too, Mom," I said.

"I have to go, okay? I'm going to make a phone call," she said.

"Okay."

About two days after my mother made a phone call I was given a new mattress. The case manager himself came down to assist the situation. I was chained up to the come along, and caseworker Brutis had me stand outside my cell. The case manager gave me a new mattress, and he threw the old one away.

"Okay, Bower," he said. "You should be all set."

I was placed back into my cell, and the correctional staff forgot to replace my sheets.

"What about my bedding?"

I tried to grab their attention.

"Hey, excuse me," I said. "What about my bedding?"

No one cared to answer me.

I noticed the staff began to start showers, and they had the come along with them. The correctional staff started yard too. Brutis and Gross went cell to cell for showers and cell to cell for yards. The correctional staff would take inmates out to yard first thing in the morning. Once an inmate was outside, they were only given one hour for yard. The shower was different in a few ways. With the shower, inmates received only fifteen minutes, but some staff were lenient on this entire idea. Not all of the time because most of the staff wanted us to hurry. They wanted us to be done on their watch. As I was in my cell, Brutis came up to my door.

"Yard, Bower?"

"Ya," I said.

"Okay, get ready," he said. "I will be back in five minutes."

I waited those five minutes for him to return. Once he did, he directed me to strip, and I had to become fully naked. He asked me to bend over and spread

342

my cheeks. Then he asked me to open my mouth and stick out my tongue. The entire thing was very uncomfortable, and I hated it very much. I then dressed myself in my orange jumpsuit and my orange shoes. After that I was restrained in the come along, and I was escorted to the yard. While I was outside, I began pacing back and forth. A man named Jeff Johnson was placed next to me. He was black, and he had a shaved head. He had brown eyes and many tattoos on his arms. Jeff Johnson was in for murder, and he was ruthless. He bragged about how he murdered a white woman. Him being black didn't bother me, but what bothered me was his racism. I couldn't stand a racist black person. They stood for what was righteous in the Civil Rights era. However back then black men and women had it very difficult growing up. I have no idea how hard it was for them. Nevertheless, it gives no one the right to murder another person then turn around and say they did it because of what they went through. That is exactly what he did. It was distasteful and disturbing to my ears. I couldn't even look at him with respect. Plus it was a woman he murdered. That women was probably a mother, and she probably had children.

"I killed that white bitch," he said. "I would do it again in a heartbeat too."

"You're evil," I said. "You have your entire life to think about what you did."

"Fuck you," he said.

343

"No fuck you," I said. "I don't want to hear about how you murdered someone."

Jeff Johnson began to spit through the fence, and I lifted my arm up to protect my face. He spit right on my cheek, and he caught me right under my glasses. I was thankful that he didn't hit me in the eye. I went back inside after my hour was up, and I waited for lunch to arrive. The meals came on a big metal cart, and the cart had locks on the sides. The correctional staff opened the cart doors and gathered the trays. Then they began to stick the trays onto a small rolling cart. The staff delivered the trays one cell at a time. The kitchen provided tea with each meal, except during breakfast because during breakfast we were given two cups of coffee. The coffee was always cold, or at least lukewarm. The days went by slow, but in reality they also went by fast. Think about it for a moment, just because I'm locked up, doesn't mean time stops. It keeps going, and in the community people live busy lives. I also realized I couldn't make it on the protective custody unit. I was so used to being confined in segregation. Plus being autistic and in prison doesn't really go hand in hand. I feared for my safety, and I was very vulnerable to other inmates. But the administration wanted me to try it again, and so they placed me back on A-unit.

"Mr. Bower," Duke said, "I need to speak with you."

"Okay," I said.

I walked up to my cell door, and he pulled up a chair. I used my toilet as a chair, and he used a plastic red chair to sit on.

"We are going to give A-unit another shot," he said. "Now we can't keep giving you chances like this. If you don't do well, you will be put back on administrative confinement. Do you understand?"

I looked at him in his eyes.

"Yes sir," I said.

"Then sign this form," he said.

After I signed the form, he left, and three hours later I was sent to Alpha unit.

Chapter 32 Back to A-Unit

The sign of autism in adults are as followed: 3 Lack of interest in sharing enjoyment, interests, and achievements with other people.

I was back on A-unit, and as I arrived everyone was locked down in their cells. I was escorted by caseworker Johndis to my cell, and she unlocked the cell door for me. I went into my new cell, and she closed the door behind me. My new celly had pictures of women in bikinis on the wall. They were wearing blue bikinis and black bikinis. The pictures looked to be cut out from a magazine. There were multiple photos of women bending over and revealing their breasts. I noticed some were actresses and others were models. It was very tempting to look at because the women were very attractive. All the women who worked here were fat and ugly. It was very difficult to have any emotion for them at all. I believed I could make do with my new celly. I didn't feel afraid, and he seemed to be pretty relaxed. He was white, and his hair was red.

"What's up?"

"Not much," I said.

"You have top bunk," he said.

The cell was small, and I wasn't sure how other inmates did it. How they survived one another.

"If you have to use the toilet, I have a set up for that," he said.

He stood up and showed me a sheet. The sheet hooked into the wall like a curtain.

"You take this sheet, and you spread it out," he said. "Then you hook it into the wall."

He was pointing at a small metal hook in the wall. I noticed he probably designed the hook himself.

"I see," I said.

"Pretty clever, huh?" he said. "So what's your name?"

"I'm Austin," I said.

"Well Austin, I'm Red. They call me Red because of my hair."

"So Red, when is canteen?"

"It's on every Wednesday," he said. "You turn your canteen slip in on Sunday nights."

"When do we go out to yard?"

"Well, we go out every day for one hour," he said. "And there are soda pop machines outside too, so you can buy a soda if you pay for soda tokens."

"Okay," I said.

"Also we go to the day hall for forty-five minutes each day," he said.

"Okay."

Red had a baseball game on his television. It appeared to be the Chicago Cubs playing the Boston Red Sox.

"Do you like baseball?"

"A little," I said. "I am more of a football kind of guy."

"Ya, well take a load off and relax," he said.

I was watching Red's television, and the game was at Fenway Park. I began to feel uneasy for some reason, and I started to feel uncomfortable. I think I was claustrophobic, and the tight quarters of confinement made me feel uneasy. I really hated it, and I wanted out. All of a sudden, an alarm went off, and the alarm was near Red's bed. Red turned his alarm off and stood up quickly.

"Time for chow," Red said.

Caseworker Johndis was standing at the control sector. Johndis opened a locked box and began pressing a digital screen. The digital buttons controlled the cell doors. One door popped after the other, and I went to chow with the protective custody group. We walked the hallway and passed the law library room. I looked into the legal library, and I saw computers and books. I also saw four large bookshelves, and the bookshelves had hundreds of books waiting to be read. There were two separate rooms in the legal library. One of those rooms was for the legal research, and I also saw a typewriter. The legal library was on the left of me. As I continued to walk, I passed the main library. The main library was very large, and classes for GED testing happened in the main library. I saw many bookshelves and computers, and I also saw seven long tables. I entered the door that led to the chow hall, and I took my place in line. I grabbed my food, and I took a seat. The whole thing reminded me of high school again. How I would get my food tray and find a seat to sit at with other students to socialize. However, this was different, and I knew that it was different. This was more dangerous than high school. I was in prison, and these weren't students.

A-unit had four sections to it.

The sections were A-1 wing, A-2 wing, A-2 center, and A-1 center.

In each section the inmates were all separated from one another. A-1 wing stuck with only A-1 wing, and that meant eating, and yard, and day hall activities.

A-2 wing stuck with A-2 wing for activities, and the list goes on.

Misconduct reports were written on inmates who chose to cross to other units. It was designed that way to protect other inmates from fights and things of that nature. When breakfast, lunch, and supper were called, inmates came out assigned to their group. Breakfast began with A-1 wing, and once their entire group exited, A-1 center would follow. From there the list went on. Once chow was over, the sergeant called for A-1 wing to leave. Then the sergeant called for A-1 center. The sergeant eventually made his way to A-2 wing and wrapped up chow.

I was headed back to my cell to lock down, and I couldn't handle being on the unit anymore. I had a very difficult time being isolated with another man. I hated it, and I couldn't stand it any more. I felt like I was in danger, and I wanted to return to the mental health unit. I wanted to receive mental health services for treatment. The administration kept denying my return, and I couldn't do anything about it. I felt like killing myself on a daily basis. I had already experienced quite a lot of trauma, and I wanted out. My mind was cloudy, and I couldn't think straight. The more I thought about it, the more I fought against it. The thoughts were very overwhelming, and they raced through my mind. I felt very unsafe, so I began to pound on my cell door.

"Hey caseworker! Please, somebody help me," I said.

I began to pound on the door even more.

"Caseworker!"

350

"Are you okay?" Red asked me while he was seated on his bunk.

"Hey someone," I said.

"What's wrong, Austin?"

"I feel like dying," I said. "I feel like killing myself."

"What are they going to help you with?"

"I don't know," I said. "I want to go back to the mental health unit."

I had my head turned slightly while I spoke to Red.

"Hey! Someone help me," I said. "Caseworker!"

I saw a caseworker walking in my direction.

"What do you want, Bower?"

"I'm going to kill myself," I said.

Smith walked down the steps and came to my cell door.

"What's that?"

"I'm going to kill myself," I said.

"Why?"

"Because I want to die," I said.

"But why do you want to die?"

"Because I hate it here," I said.

"Okay," he said. "I will have an escort come and get you."

351

Smith walked away and got on his radio. I heard him call for an escort. About five minutes later an escort arrived at the spin door. He walked with Smith to my cell door.

"Put your hands behind your back," he said.

I did as he asked, and the escort placed me in handcuffs. I survived A-unit for three days, which was a record for me. My escort was black, and he wore glasses. He led me up the stairs and off of A-unit.

Chapter 33 The Control Unit

The sign of autism in adults are as followed: 4 The lack of empathy or understanding.

I was in the control unit naked, and I had nothing in my cell. I had no bunk, and I had no bed to lay on. I was given a green smock to wear, and it had Velcro straps on the back of it. I was in cell sixteen again, and I didn't know if I would survive.

"Hey Bower," Kenn said.

Kenn was yelling through his cell door. His cell was straight across from mine. Kenn was short and stubby with red hair. He claimed to be Native American, but he was white and his eyes were blue.

"Isn't it true that you got fucked by Navajo?" he said.

"That's not true," I said. "That's not true at all."

"Ya right," Kenn said. "Put that on something."

"What the hell does that mean? Put that on something. You sound stupid.

"If it's not true," he said, "then swear it on your mom."

"No," I said. "But it's not true."

"No one believes you, Bower," he said. "You got fucked."

"Shut up," I said. "Leave me alone."

"Hey Bower," Kenn said. "Why don't you lay on the ground? I'm sure it feels good."

"Shut up," I said.

"No," he said. "I'm going to fuck with you all day."

I took my smock, and I put it under my head for a pillow. As I laid on the floor, I tried to get comfortable, but that was near impossible. I was far from comfortable, and my side was in pain. I tossed and I turned on the cement floor. I chose to stand up, and even my feet were in pain. I knew the process to get my belongings back, mainly because I've been here before, and I knew the struggle it was. The days drug out in the control unit, and I was in pain every minute of it. Kenn was a young punk, and all he wanted was to be accepted. He tried to hang with bigger gangs, and he claimed to be a blood. I knew he was a fake though. I have never met a Native American with blue eyes in my entire life. He would tease me, and he would call me names. He would tell me to kill myself and that I should hang myself with my green smock. He would give me ideas to cut my arms with razors. I almost gave in to his temptations, and I had every reason to. I was in hell, and the earth left me a long time ago. Each day drug out with brand new problems. I dreaded waking up every day, and I hoped that one day I wouldn't wake up.

I took showers when showers were called, and I cleaned my cell every Saturday. The guard would bring around the cleaning cart and give cleaning supplies to the inmates. I wasn't allowed to use the spray bottle. No one was allowed to use the spray bottle. I figured I was going to be down here for a while. I just knew it, and the thought of it paralyzed me and my thinking. I didn't ever leave the unit unless I had a visit. There was nothing else to it. If my family didn't show, I didn't receive a visit. I had my Bible to read, but believe me my faith was falling apart. I wondered how much longer of this I could take before I gave up the idea of Jesus. I prayed, but nothing would happen. Even know nothing would happen for me, I would still pray. I prayed for my family all the time. I prayed that good things would happen in their lives. I sure knew nothing good was happening in my life. Being in this environment caused me to lash out. I would hold my tray, and I wouldn't give my tray back. I went mentally insane, and everything got the best of me. I watched one inmate throw urine on a guard through his hatch. He also refused to give his tray back, and after that the guards beat him down. I waited nearly three months before I was moved cells. I hated cell sixteen because of the camera, and there was no privacy in my cell. It took me two months to get my bunk back. After I earned everything back, I was moved to another cell. I was moved to cell eight, and it sucked. The last inmate that was in cell eight wiped his poop all over the walls. A team of staff had to clean the walls while wearing white pullover jumpsuits. The smell was disturbing. No one cared though, and I knew they didn't care.

So I told the correctional staff I was suicidal, which started me all over to square one. I was moved back to cell sixteen a short time after. I had to start the entire process all over again. I don't know if it was stupid or wise. Regardless of what it was, I needed to be able to breathe, and I couldn't breathe in that cell. So in a way I did what was best for me. Another month went by like nothing, and I had nothing to show for it. When I realized segregation was torture on many levels, I chose to flood my cell. I had clothing, such as a shirt and a jumpsuit, the normal stuff, and I flushed them all down the toilet. I flushed the toilet for over twenty minutes, and no one knew about it. The guards were in their office sitting on their asses. The water began to flow out like a river bank breaking. The water accumulated and washed out evenly throughout the control unit. The water began to go under cell doors, and it washed under the gate too.

"Bower, what the hell!" Burns came out of the office yelling. He was wearing a blue state uniform.

"Holy shit," Copley said.

"Go fuck yourselves," I said. "I want out of this

cell."

"You're not going anywhere," Burns said.

I watched as a team of seven correctional officers cleaned up the overflow of water. I ended up receiving three misconduct reports, and I had to restart my cell time. I knew that I shouldn't of done it, and it was a poor choice on my part. Nevertheless, I felt so obligated to act out. I was in a bad situation, and I knew an injustice when I saw one. I had lots of good time that I had to earn back. I was angry because of how much segregation time I already did. I had to start from scratch now with everything, and my family just wanted me out. I was prolonging my opportunities in life. I only acted out because I couldn't handle the problems that laid before me. I was in need of true help, and I was dead inside. I felt like my life was worth absolutely nothing. My family could not help me, and I was helpless. I slumped and struggled through the next three months of mental warfare. My limbs physically felt heavy, and I couldn't even do one push up. I was gaining weight again and losing heart. Nevertheless, I eventually moved cells. I was moved from cell sixteen to cell nine. This time the cell smelled better, and it didn't smell like shit. I stayed in cell nine for quite some time. You see the case manager for the control had a list. The list was known as the move up list. The list had three inmates on it at all times. The best behaved inmate was the first to move up, and the inmate who fit the right criteria was moved up first.

Chapter 34 Back to C-Unit

Some causes that form autism are as followed: 1 The lack of oxygen at birth. 2 Chemical imbalance at birth. 3 Viruses at birth. 4 Rubella other wise known as (German Measles) while the mother is pregnant.

I ignored the other inmates with the best of my abilities. I also didn't forget about the oath I made to God. I made a strong, powerful oath to never return to prison. My oath to God was sincere and honest from my heart. I wanted changes to happen in my life. Good changes, and that started with me. I ignored, ignored, and ignored some more. There was no textbook on how to do it. There was only me, and what I had to do for my survival. Every day was hard without a shadow of a doubt. It was the most difficult thing I had to go through. Prison was designed to be rough and tough. It was designed to break you or make you. I thought it made everyone worse and caused a lot of bad effects to others and their families.

"Bower, you're moving to C-unit," Copley said.

He gave me a plastic bag through the hatch, and I waited for my escort to arrive. I was escorted by Officer Gunner. He was black and had a low trimmed haircut. His walk was one of those walks a movie star would have. He showed no fear, and he was tough. You could see it all over him. He had a large, strong chest and swollen arms. He looked like a football player of sorts, almost like a utility man. Someone who could play every spot of the field. He had a low baritone voice; his voice was almost identical to Stevie Wonder. I wouldn't be surprised if he could sing. I pictured Officer Gunner singing Wonders 1984 smash hit "I just called to say I love you." I mean I never heard the guy sing, but I wouldn't be surprised if he could. Gunner escorted me into the elevator and through the hallway. He received permission to walk me to C-unit on his radio.

"Hey Gunner, what's good?"

Caseworker Crock caught his attention. Crock was standing outside of C-unit waiting on me. I was in full body chain restraints.

"Not much, same old same old," Gunner said.

"How's the family?"

"You know I don't talk about family here," he said.

"My bad," Crock said.

I went through the C-unit spin door, and I was led up the stairs too.

"Bower, you're going to upper one," Crock said. "You'll have the best view in the house. You'll have the view of the whole unit."

He placed my belongings on the laundry table, and he escorted me up the steps. Then he removed my chain restraints at the door.

"Strip," he said.

I didn't argue with him. I just did as he asked. I began to unbutton my jumpsuit, and I removed my segregation shoes. I handed everything to him through the hatch, and he examined the items carefully.

"Okay," he said. "Let me see the bottom of your feet."

I lifted my heels, and he observed them.

"Okay," he said. "Now lift up your balls."

I did as he asked.

"Now turn around and spread your ass," he said.

I complied to all his orders.

"Okay," he said. "Let me see the inside of your mouth."

I did everything as he asked, and I also assumed he was gay. I only say that because every other male officer wants to get through the strip search quickly, but not him. It was very strange to me to have that experience.

I went to lay down on my mattress. The boat was

gray, and the mattress was yellow. I waited while the case workers searched through all of my belongings. I stood at my cell door watching them as they did. The inmate porters were out roaming around. They were in charge of the laundry and the cleaning of the showers. Also from what I was told, the caseworkers were no longer able to work with the food, mainly because there were reports of them spitting in the tea. There were also reports of them doing unethical things with the food. So the Lincoln Correctional Center administration had to find a solution, and so they did. They made the porters in charge of the food. It used to not be that way when I first started doing my sentence.

I was waiting for my items, and I was standing by my door still. I was doing this because I didn't trust the inmates who were working near my items. I didn't trust anybody at all. My heart became hardened over time and desensitized. I really had no feeling, and I didn't feel anything. Like I was emotionless and careless to emotion. I didn't care who lived or died, and I didn't care who didn't care for me. I also didn't care for someone who did care for me. I had been beaten psychologically and emotionally to where life itself did not matter to me. I had pent up rage inside of me, and it was held back. It was the only way I would make it out. I held everything back, even though the injustice was right in front of me. Nevertheless there were those who would say I'm just a *criminal* or a *monster*. It's not like I was a murderer though. I was around monsters, and murderers, and people who did evil things. I had to live with inmates who stabbed people to death and inmates who raped innocent women and children. I was living with ungodly human beings.

"Bower, you have a clergy visit," Crock said.

I saw my belongings on the table, and that worried me. I had a visit, and I didn't have my belongings yet. All of this worried me because I didn't want any of my items to be stolen. I had a radio, and I had a television, and books. I had a lot of things that I was worried about.

"Do you want to go?"

The question was a hard one to answer, but I had to make up my mind. I had an intuition telling me not go, but I decided to go anyway.

"Ya, I'll go," I said.

"Okay, I'll bring you your khakis," he said.

I waited for him to gather my brown khakis and my boots.

He radioed for an escort and grabbed the full body chain restraints. I noticed that the porters had to lock down before I came out of my cell. I was greeted by an escort and placed in full body chain restraints, and I was escorted to visiting.

Chapter 35 Gut Feeling

Asperger's Syndrome is a mild form of autism, and is listed as one of the disorders in (ASD) Autsim Spectrum Disorder.

I looked at my clergy visitor for a moment, and I knew right off the bat he wasn't who I hoped he would be. He was brown, and he wore glasses. His name was Pastor Zenock, and he was nearing his late fifties. I was hoping for someone else, but he didn't show. The person who I wanted to see was a friend. A friend who took care of me when I was younger. I used to live in a group home, and I had a person who cared for me. Well this wasn't him, and right then I knew I shouldn't of showed up. I had a bad feeling that my belongings would be stolen. It went through my head over and over again.

"Austin," he said, "how are you doing?"

"I'm not doing very well," I said.

"What part of the Bible would you like to read?"

I looked his direction, and then I looked away for a moment.

"Hey, can I go back?"

The question caught my visitor by surprise.

"Sure," he said.

My visitor stepped out of the room and asked the officers if I could go back. The officers came my direction and opened the door.

"You want to go back, Bower?"

"Yes," I said.

"All right, let's go," he said.

I was happy I didn't have to deal with Floos, and that made things much better for me. Word has it he became a caseworker. I hoped I wouldn't have to see him anytime soon. I stripped out for the male officer, and I had an escort walk me back to my unit. As I arrived the porter inmates went to lock down. I noticed my items were all gone, which scared me a little. I was escorted up the stairs and to my cell door. I looked in my cell, and all my belongings were on the floor in my cell. My television was on the desk, and it appeared that everything was okay. The caseworker removed my chains and strip searched me. Afterwards I was left in my cell. I went to inspect my items, and I had a bad feeling about something. I noticed that my radio was gone, and I also noticed the thing that bothered me the most. My television, my television had a scratch going all the way through the LED screen. I was outraged, and I looked out my window. I saw the two porters laughing and giving each other high fives. The worst part about all this was the fact that the caseworkers allowed it to happen. I had no idea what to do, and I was saddened already. I had been through so much trauma as it was. I didn't need this, I thought, and it drove me mad. I went to the corner of my cell because I saw a bag. The bag was full of yellow urine. I was able to smell it before I knew where it was located. The urine was all over my pillow. I went to the corner of my cell, and I cried for a long time. I had my head down, and my head was in my hands. I was crying tears of pain, and I had no one to tell. Who would care? It would be days before I could use the phone. The porter who did it came up to my cell mopping the floor. He looked into my cell and began to talk trash to me.

"Hey punk, that's what you get," he said. "Is the little baby crying?"

He was mocking me now, and making fun of me.

"Leave me alone," I said.

"Is the baby crying?"

"Leave me alone," I said.

He mocked some more.

"Hey caseworker! Caseworker!"

I began to yell repeatedly

"You're a fucking snitch," he said.

I walked up to my cell door, and the caseworker was standing near the stair rails.

"What's going on?"

366

He was looking at my cell.

"He was making fun of me," I said.

"That's what you called me for?"

"Ya," I said.

"Go lay down, Bower," he said.

"No, he was making fun of me," I said.

"Ya, we'll take care of it," he said. "Go relax."

I didn't believe him at all, and I had no reason to. I cleaned up the urine before I laid down. I used my shampoo to clean the wall and my boat. Then I took off my pillowcase, and then I put a shirt over the pillow. I also dumped the urine out into the toilet, and I flushed the bag with it. The toilet was strong enough to pull the small plastic bag all the way under. I took my belongings and organized them all. I took my television, and I hooked it up to the wall jack. I was angry every time I looked at my television, but what was I to do? There was nothing that I could do but accept it. So I did, and I rolled with the punches of what just happened. I also knew that I was hated very much, and they really had no reason to hate me. I never did anything to them for them to hate me. I know one thing, and that is I should trust my gut instinct. I need to trust myself more, I thought. I used this as a learning curve in my life.

Chapter 36 Seeing Hawkboy

Here are five symptomes in Asperger's as followed: 1 Anxiety Disorder. 2 Obsessive-compulsive disoder (OCD). 3 Nonverbal learning disorder. 4 Social anxiety disorder. 5 Depression.

"Mr. Bower," Duke said.

He was standing on the other side of my door.

"I received your request about your good time," he said. "We approved it. You have had no misconduct reports for a full year. You should be proud."

"Thank you," I said.

"Thank yourself, Mr. Bower," he said. "You're the one doing the work."

I studied Duke over carefully.

"You will be out of here next month," he said.

"Okay," I said.

"Keep in mind that you have twenty-eight days left."

"Yes, sir," I said.

"So don't fuck it up."

"I won't," I said.

"Because if you do, your last six months will go out

the window. If the administration approves you, you will be out in twenty-eight days," he said.

"Okay," I said. "Thank you for explaining that to me."

"No problem," he said. "In twenty-eight days you might be gone."

"See you later, Mr. Bower."

Duke began to walk away while he used his cane. I went to lay down on my bunk and watched some television. I was watching Judge Judy, and she was schooling some teen for breaking some kid's angel. The angel was made of glass, and the teen was holding his broken angel in his hands. He was showing the cameras the broken angel. The teen said he received the angel as a Christmas gift. I wish I had my own television show, I thought while I was watching him talk. I imagined being on television, and explaining to an audience what prison does to the brain. How segregation conflicts the mind and damages the nerves. I wasn't sure this was proven, but one could only think. Prison is a dangerous place to be, and it was a harsh environment to be in. Two caseworkers came to my cell, and one of them was holding the come along.

"Yard, Bower?" Gross asked.

"Ya, I'll go to yard," I said.

I was taken to yard by Gross and Johndis. I was led

down the stairs and through the yard door. Johndis
uncuffed me once I was in the cage. Johndis then
locked the cage after she locked the hatch. Johndis
and Gross went back inside. There were three
sections to each unit. There were three yard sections
for C-1 and three yard sections for C-2. There were a
total of six sections. Each section held one inmate
during segregation yard time. I watched the C-1
correctional staff bring inmates out from C-1 unit.
The C-1 officers were Brutis and Lock. The inmate
they had with them was Hawkboy.

"Bower," he said. "Is that you?"

He recognized me right away.

"What do you want?"

I was leaning against the fence.

"I want to talk you," he said.

"Why?"

Brutis was locking Hawkboy into the cage. After
Brutis and Lock finished securing Hawkboy, they
both went back inside.

"You lied, Austin," he said.

"Says who? You?"

I was pacing back and forth now.

"You are no one to call a liar," I said. "You lied to
me. The crazy thing is, you ruined my life."

"Fuck you and your life," he said.

"I'm here when I shouldn't be," I said. "My attorney told me you took a plea. You took a plea before I did."

"Fuck you," he said.

"I'm not afraid of you," I said. "I don't fear you."

"Well you should," he said.

"You're a coward," I said. "You take advantage of people like me."

"You're a dead man walking," he said. "Once I get out, I am going to kill you."

"You're just mad I got probation, and you didn't," I said.

"You got probation?" he said. "I'm definitely gonna kill you."

"I am not afraid of you," I said.

"I'm going to stab you," he said.

"Why are you mad at me?"

I was holding the fence with my hands up high.

"You took a plea bargain before I did," I said. "And I still got probation."

I could tell that made him angry.

"Motherfucker," he said.

"You told on me, Hawkboy," I said. "And I didn't even do the crime. You were only caught because you lost your shoe. And you're the reason why other inmates hate me. You spread lies and make things up. Yet you have no paperwork on me. Plus you refused to appeal your paperwork. All because you ratted me out. Why would you want to hide your statement?"

He was quiet for a moment.

"I'm done talking to you," he said.

He was pacing back and forth now.

"You are a dead man walking," he said. "I am going to kill you."

"I don't care what you do," I said.

After that I kept ignoring him, and I minded my own business. I waited for the staff to take me inside. So I sat on the ground, and eventually Johndis and Gross returned. I was cuffed to the come along and taken inside.

Chapter 37 The Toilet Man

I was standing at my cell door because I had nothing else to do. That is when I witnessed the correctional staff move my neighbor. The neighbor I had was easy to get along with. He didn't yell through the vent or bang on the wall to keep me awake at night. The neighbor I had was replaced with the toilet man. Everyone called him the toilet man. His real name was Kelsy Baker. He was tall and old. He had gray hair and long limber arms. He had angered many other inmates by flushing his toilet repeatedly in the early morning hours. Kelsy was like me; he had a green light on him too. He angered the wrong inmates by flushing his toilet while they were sleeping. I knew this would be bad. I also thought this was an idea brought up by the administration. Kelsy didn't say much, and he wasn't a talker. He ran his toilet instead of running his mouth.

I watched as the guards unchained Kelsy. I could see them through the left side of my window. The chains made a clashing sound as they hit the floor. In my mind I thought how awful it would be to get hit with those chains. The guards secured Baker into his cell, and I slowly walked back to my mattress. Nothing happened the first twenty minutes, but I knew something would happen soon. I knew because of the stories I heard during yard. I was laying down, and then it began.

"Flush!"

I thought, okay he only did it once, nothing to be worried about.

"Flush!"

He did it a second time, and I still hoped that would be it.

"Flush!"

My hopes were soon dismissed.

"Flush, flush, flush, flush, flush, flush, flush, flush!"

"Knock that shit off," I said.

"Flush!"

"Hey Baker, knock that shit off," I said.

I began to pace back and forth in my cell, and I was angry.

"Flush, flush, flush!"

This can't be, I thought. I am doing so good, and I am almost out of here. I am getting so close to being released. Why would anyone want to do this to me? I sat down at my desk, and I began to write a letter to my mother. I grabbed my blue pen, and I found a piece of lined paper. I began to tell my mother everything. I told her every thing about Baker and the administration. What I hated about the mail system was the fact I couldn't seal my mail. It was policy that the correctional staff received the mail unsealed. With legal mail I could seal, but not with mail going to family. In the past I witnessed the correctional officers read other inmates' mail. I watched them take the mail out of the brown box and read it. I soon became discouraged, and I realized there was nothing my mother could do. I put the pen down, and I went to my mattress. I laid down on my mattress looking at the ceiling, almost as if I could see through it to heaven. I began to pray to God to help understand why this was happening.

"God, why is this happening? I know you are a God of mercy, so why is this happening to me? I did nothing wrong to deserve this, God. Please explain to me what is happening," I prayed.

I continued to look up to the ceiling for answers. Meanwhile Baker continued to flush the toilet over and over again. I hoped he wouldn't do it at night, but I knew what hope was. Hope was something that we couldn't see. Hope was an invisible force, and that force was only there when we least expected it. I knew it was up to me to ignore Baker to avoid any trouble from him. I was beginning to earn my good time back one month at a time. I believed this administration knew I was nearing a discharge and that they wanted me to stay. They pulled all the stops from the metal table from the long amounts of segregation time to the visiting staff assaulting me and now this. I had no idea when all of this was going to end. I had a clue though, and that was once I discharged. Once discharged everything would be better. I would be safer and secure in a new environment. Little did I know about culture shock and reentering the community after years of my life spent in solitary confinement. I knew nothing of the sort; however, I had a taste of culture shock with my probation situation. I was so used to being confined into a cell that once I received probation I was in shock of my surroundings.

"Flush!"

The noise of the toilet brought me back to reality. It was annoying more than it was loud. I mean, don't get me wrong, it was loud, but it being annoying was worse.

"Flush, flush, flush, flush, flush!"

"Hey Baker, why don't you flush yourself down the toilet?" I said.

"Flush!"

I rose off of my mattress, and I stood on my toilet.

"Hey motherfucker," I said. "Why don't you flush yourself down the toilet?"

"Fuck you, punk," Baker said.

"Oh, he speaks," I said. "What else do you have to say?"

"Kill yourself, punk," he said.

"No, you kill yourself, mother fucker," I said.

"Flush, flush, flush, flush, flush!"

He continued to flush his toilet all the way until dinnertime. I ate my dinner, and then I turned in my tray, and Baker was back at it again.

"Flush, flush, flush!"

I had my headphones on, and I laid on my mattress thinking this couldn't be real. However, it was real, and it wasn't going to stop. The administration wanted me to mess up, but I couldn't give them that satisfaction. So I dealt with it like a soldier would. I prayed night after night that Baker would soon be moved. He continued to flush his toilet for an entire week, and it was getting old fast. It was old the very first day he started doing all of this. Nevertheless, it didn't matter when he started; all that mattered to me is when he would stop. He wasn't stopping anytime soon, and the noise was getting to me.

"Flush, flush, flush, flush, flush!"

"Come on man, it's been one week," I said. "Give it a rest."

"Fuck you, punk," he said.

"Flush, flush, flush, flush, flush, flush, flush!"

The day would carry on into the night, and all I heard was flushing. His name was the toilet man for a reason. He did this to everyone, and everyone he did it to hated him. He must of did this to the wrong Mexican, I thought. He probably pissed off a MS13 gang member or something. Everyone knew Kelsy Baker had a green light on him. Fuck this motherfucker, I thought. It was nighttime, and all the lights were out. I stood up on the toilet, and I began to talk trash to Baker.

"Hey Baker," I said.

"Hey, you piece of shit."

"Wake up, motherfucker," I said. "You aren't going to sleep. Wake your ass up."

I knew Baker was asleep because he hadn't flushed the toilet for the past two hours.

"Wake your ass up, Baker," I said.

"Flush, flush, flush, flush, flush, flush!"

"Ya, now you're awake," I said. "How does it feel, motherfucker?"

"Fuck you, punk," he said.

"No, fuck you," I said. "Now I'm going to bed."

"Flush, flush, flush, flush, flush, flush, flush!"

I laid on my mattress until I fell asleep, and eventually the noise didn't bother me anymore. Baker continued to flush his toilet for the next two weeks. Believe me, it got it to me, but I couldn't let the correctional staff know that it did. For the next two weeks, I put up with the loud, annoying noise of the toilet man. The administration figured out it wouldn't get to me. I wouldn't let it get to me. I refused to end up back in the control unit.

"Baker," Brutis said.

I could see Brutis outside of my cell window.

"Pack your things," he said. "You're going to delta unit."

The correctional worker gave Baker a plastic bag, and after about five minutes Baker was gone. I watched as Baker walked down the steps to the spine door. He was headed to the mental health unit, and I slept like a baby that night.

378

Chapter 38 The Ombudsman

I was laying on my mattress after lunch, and the caseworkers began doing yard again. I sat up and walked over to my door. As I was looking out the window, the correctional workers were approaching my cell door. The workers were Brutis and King.

"Do you want yard, Bower?"

"Yes," I said.

"Okay, strip out then," he said.

I began to undress, and I took my time doing it. I looked out my cell door and noticed Brutis had a large zit on his forehead. It was white and full of puss. It was pretty disgusting if you ask me. After Brutis searched me for weapons and homemade shanks, he placed the come along handcuffs around my hands. Brutis opened my door, and King led behind us.

"It's a nice day," Brutis said. "Too bad you have to spend it in here."

"Ya, I know," I said.

"Well, let's get you some fresh air," he said.

Brutis led me out to the small yard compound and placed me in one of the segregation yard sections. I began to pace back and forth in the section. The sky was blue, and the air was peaceful. I was the only one in the yard compound, and I decided to take a seat on the ground. I picked up pebbles and tossed them with my fingers. As I was seated, I saw someone coming down the unit stairs. I didn't recognize him at first, and he was wearing civilian clothing. He was black, and he had thick eyebrows. He came outside from the yard door and approached me.

"Hello Austin," Havis said. "It's good to see you. You're almost out."

Havis was standing in front of me. Kelly Havis was the Nebraska State Ombudsman, and he had a shaved head. He was wearing a blue baseball cap to cover his head from the sun.

"Ya, I know," I said.

"How do you feel about it?"

"I'm not sure," I said. "I feel like I lost my mind a long time ago from all these years stuck in isolation."

"You've had it rough," he said. "The good news is you have only fourteen days left."

"How do you know that?"

He had a smile on his face.

380

"Because I spoke to the director myself," he said.

"So it was all approved?"

I returned the smile.

"Yes," he said.

"So I received it all back?"

I asked again because I wanted to be certain due to all the surprises that I've experienced during my sentence.

"Yes," he said.

I threw my hands in the air and began to dance. It was the first time that I really felt alive.

"So how do you feel?" he asked while adjusting his baseball cap.

"I feel great," I said.

"Good," he said. "You keep feeling great."

"Okay," I said. "I mean I will."

"Okay, I got to go," he said. "You take care, Austin."

Mr. Havis left through the yard door, and the yard door led to the unit. As I looked up at the sky I smiled. I was soon escorted back to my cell from yard, and I felt a burden lift from my shoulders.

Chapter 39 Discharge

With in three years of being released 37 percent of inmates with mental illness are locked up again. Compared to 30 percent of those who do not have mental illness.

I woke up on the day of my discharge, and I couldn't believe it was really here. The day was October 20th, 2014. I thought this day would never come because I thought I would die in prison. I sat up on my mattress while Brutis began to pass out breakfast. I stood up to receive my tray. Brutis was at my hatch, and he was staring at me.

"Bower," Brutis said, "You might as well not even eat. You can get something way better at home."

"That's true," I said.

"So do you want the tray?"

The inmate porter was holding the tray in his hands. I looked at both of them briefly.

"No, it's okay," I said.

"Are you sure?"

"Ya, I'm sure," I said.

Brutis walked away with the food porter. They both

found their way downstairs and began passing out trays. I could hear each time Brutis unlocked a hatch. I went to my mattress, and I began watching the morning news. The news wasn't talking about anything special. The only thing the news was talking about was Obamacare. The news was addressing how the affordable care act was a horrible plan. As I was watching the news, I became anxious because I was discharging from segregation. I was given no tools for the community. I spent my entire sentence in segregation, and I wasn't ready to be let out. I had no formal social practice with other inmates. I wasn't on a unit with inmates to socialize with. What I needed was not given to me. I needed to be on the mental health unit for a solid transition. I was also on a medication that did very little for me. Since I was given a false diagnosis, Dr. Pretzel gave me the wrong medication. He also stole my dignity by denying my autism and by keeping me in segregation for so many years. Even in the county jail they kept me in segregation. I spent over five years in segregation altogether, and you can't come back from that. Once you go through it, you simply can't come back from it. I hated these mental health workers for what they did to me. I wanted to see them die. They took taxpayer money and used it to beat me. They beat me psychologically, emotionally, and physically. I waited patiently to discharge, so I could soon be with my family. I was angry at the system, and I was angry at Hawkboy. I never wanted

383

to see Hawkboy again.

I was in my cell standing at my door, and I was looking out my window. Brutis had Hawkboy in full body chain restraints.

"Where's he at?"

Caseworker Brutis pointed up at my cell, and Hawkboy looked my direction. Hawkboy was in an orange jumpsuit, and he looked angry.

"You're a dead man walking," Hawkboy said. "You're a dead man walking, Bower. I'm going to kill you once I get out."

I didn't respond, and I wanted this nightmare to be over. This was a tactic by the administration because they didn't want to see me leave. I went to my mattress to lay down until it was time for me to leave. I laid on my mattress, and I was thinking about what just happened.

"I knew this administration was crooked," I said.

I was speaking to myself under my breath. I stood up, off of my mattress, and I began to pack my belongings. I started with all of my hygiene supplies and my books. I also packed my magazines and my batteries. Then I organized all of my paperwork and placed everything in a large manila folder. Next I began to unhook my television.

As I was unhooking my television, my cable input broke. It completely came out of its socket. I began to wonder why this just happened. It happened right before I was leaving. I thought about how it served its purpose, and I also thought about how God works in mysterious ways.

"Bower," Brutis said.

He didn't look happy when he called my name.

"Pack up your shit," he said. "You're leaving in five minutes."

"Can I get a plastic bag?"

"Ya, I'll get you one," he said.

Brutis walked to the main office, and he grabbed me a plastic bag. Brutis walked up the stairs and came to my cell door. He unlocked my hatch, and he gave me a large plastic bag. I took the bag, and I packed all my belongings. Then I rolled up my blankets and sheets, and I stood at my door. I stood there waiting patiently for the moment to happen. I knew that my mother was waiting for me, and I was waiting for her.

"You ready. Bower?"

"Yes," I said.

Brutis was holding the full body chain restraints in his hands. He had another caseworker assist him, and he opened my hatch with his keys.

"Place your hands through the hatch," he said. "You know the drill."

I placed my hands through the hatch, and he placed the cuffs on me. He made sure that the cuffs were tight. Then Brutis opened the cell door.

"Face the door, Bower," Brutis said.

Brutis began to place the belly chain around my waist, and then he moved to the leg irons. Once he was all finished, he shut the cell door.

"Let's go," Brutis said.

"Bye bitch," Jeff Johnson said.

He was giving me the middle finger.

"Fuck you, faggot," Kogill said.

He was on the bottom tier, and he still had six years left. I was walking down the steps from my cell door, and I headed to the spin door. Brutis opened the spin door, and he escorted me through the hallway. As I walked the hallway, I saw Hawkboy in the segregation yard. I could see him through the hallway window. I went past all of Charlie unit, and then I went past all of Delta unit. Then I went past all of Echo unit. I didn't have to go past Beta unit because we took the long way. I arrived at turnkey, and I walked past the gym. Brutis led me past a locked gate and through a hallway. The hallway connected the Lincoln Correctional Center to the Diagnostic Evaluation Center. Brutis led me through two large doors, and from there Brutis led me to the hospital. Brutis pressed a big red button outside the hospital door. The door made a pop noise, and Brutis led me into the infirmary. As I walked forward, I could see the metal table. That table brought me so much pain, and to think I won't have to see it ever again. It was very rewarding to know I was leaving. Brutis walked me over to the nurse's station, and the nurse grabbed a blood pressure cuff. The nurse did all my vitals, and afterwards Brutis escorted me back through the hospital door.

"So Bower," Brutis said, "what are you going to eat?"

"Red Robin," I said.

"Really?"

"Yes," I said. "My family and me are going later today."

Brutis led me through an elevator and past a large metal door. I was led to a long desk, and it was the same long desk during my admissions. I approached two state correctional officers. They were both wearing a blue uniform with an American flag on the side of their sleeve. It was where Brutis would leave me, but before Brutis left, he removed the full body chain restraints. He began with the ankle cuffs and worked his way to the handcuffs. I was left alone at the central booking counter of the diagnostic evaluation center. The correctional officer in front of me gave me a form to sign. The form was for a one hundred dollar gate fee.

"Sign here," he said.

I signed the form he had in front of me. After I signed the form, he led me to the other side of the counter. His partner grabbed a large box and placed it in front of me.

"What size jeans?"

"46," I said.

"What size shirt?"

"2x," I said.

I was given poorly made jeans and a plaid button up shirt. He led me to a room that I could change in. This time I didn't have to strip, and it felt good to know that I didn't have to. I felt like a human being again. After I changed my outfit, the officer led me to a camera room.

"Come with me," he said. "Take a seat, and sit up straight."

I did as he asked, and he took my picture. After my photo I was led through a large door. I carried all my property with me, and the officer handed me a check. I was escorted to the lobby, and that's when everything stopped.

"Hi Mom," I said.

"Hi honey," she said.

I walked over to my mother, and I placed my belongings on the ground. My mom wrapped her arms around me, and she didn't let go. She hugged me tightly in her arms, and I didn't let go. We both stood there holding one another. It was as if the world had stopped and the moon fell from the sky. I didn't say a word, and neither did she. All she did was hold me, and she held me for a long time. My mother held me for an eternity in her arms. I was lost in the moment, and I had survived so much, and it was finally over. I knew it was over, and my mother did too.

Merry Faulson was standing in front of us while she was waiting for me to leave. She had a smile on her face, but I could see through her smile. I knew who she really was, and she wasn't my friend. The only thing that I cared about was leaving.

The day I left was a very special day, and I had family all around me. My brothers and my sisters, my mother, and my grandma, and even my nephews. I went to Red Robin to eat, and I had a juicy, large, mouth-watering burger. After Red Robin, my family and I went to the guitar center, and I played the drums. It was a special day, and it was my day. I loved every second of it, and I enjoyed the presence of my family.

"Uncle Austin's home," Adam said.

"Yes, he is," Steven said.

My brother Steven is my older brother. He is older than me by one year, and I was happy he was with me. I loved happiness, and I couldn't remember the last time I was this happy. We all sat around the dinner table eating pizza and drinking soda pop. It was beautiful, and the day was beautiful. I had everything in return that Hawkboy stole from me, and he was still in prison living his pathetic life. I was now out enjoying the triumph of victory. I made it out, and I knew it too. I looked online to find more information on Hawkboy. I found out he murdered a guy at a party with a knife. I discovered he served a decade in prison before he even met me. He did time for manslaughter charges, and I wish I would have known. My mother was near me, and she stood behind me.

"It's all in the past now," she said.

She was standing behind me while I was looking at the computer screen. I was home, and that's what mattered. With my freedom I chose to do great things.

Chapter 40 News Paper Story

Former inmate with mental disabilities struggles after four years in segregation

My story was published on August 16th, 2015. It made the front page of the Sunday Paper.

"Every day I think my brain gets worse in this cell. My hope is going thin. ... I really want help Mom. Because I really feel like there might not be any left for me. ... I'm upset with myself and the sad thing is I have to live with myself in a cell 24/7 all day only thoughts race and nothing else."

***

Austin Bower slogged through every day of his prison time. Hours stacked on hours were filled with fear then defiance, pleading then door pounding, hateful insults, assaults.

He spent three years and seven months of onerous time there, in a place where a 22-year-old man with disabilities -- a "unique cookie" someone once called him -- could not hope to adjust.

391

In letters home and to District Court Judge Paul Merritt Jr., he described incidents in which he was bullied, abused and provoked by inmates and staff.

Before 2011, when he was sentenced to prison, he had spent a couple of decades defined by aggressive outbursts, learning problems, threatening behaviors, social anxiety, tics, suicide threats and attempts.

Through those years he had been diagnosed with one thing and then another by a list of doctors and psychologists. Autism, Tourette syndrome, obsessive compulsive disorder, bipolar disorder, schizophrenia, oppositional defiant disorder, borderline personality disorder.

His disabilities most likely resulted from complications of pregnancy, said his mother, Brendamae Stinson.

The Social Security Administration defined him as disabled.

And now, after more than four years spent locked up, add post traumatic stress disorder.

His prison sentence could have been predicted, given his disabilities, his vulnerability to the influence of peers, and his list of petty crimes beginning at age 18.

Even so, many would say he didn't belong there, including the judge who sentenced him.

***

"I'm scared and worried I am going to be alone on my birthday, August 9th. I will be 23 years old. Your honor, do you think I'm fat because the guy next door to me calls me obsessed and says I'm a fat a--. That hurts my feelings."

***

Shortly after his graduation from Lincoln Southeast High School in 2009, two months before his 21st birthday, Austin admitted to police he went with Charles Eagleboy, a then 33-year-old man with a long list of convictions including manslaughter, to kick down a door, bust up a surveillance camera, enter a residence and rob a man of $103.

While on probation, Austin continued to use drugs and alcohol and commit other petty offenses.

"I didn't really know where I fit in in life, and didn't know where my future was headed. And that's when I started hanging around with just the bad crowd, and all of a sudden that led to a worse crowd, and to just a corrupt crowd. ... You let the vampire in, the vampire ain't going to leave."

He found himself back in court in front of Judge Merritt, telling him he was sorry, that the apartment he lived in at 14th and D streets was a bad place for him, that if he could remain on probation he would stay away from people who were a bad influence.

Austin's attorney Norman Langemach told Merritt: "The options are pretty well running out, and I don't have anything else that I can suggest."

He needed what was not available to him: long-term dual diagnosis treatment in a facility that would keep him isolated from the people who could take advantage of him. CenterPointe was such a program, Langemach said. But CenterPointe indicated Austin would not qualify for that particular program at that time.

"You know and I know you have special needs," the judge told Austin, "but I also know you know what's right and wrong.

"With your special needs and then under the influence of drugs, that just makes you that much more usable, if you will, by somebody else."

Probation wasn't working. And so Merritt sentenced him to prison, "no part of which shall be in solitary confinement, except for violation of prison rules."

His prison sentence started March 8, 2011. By April 1, he was pleading with prison staff for protective custody.

"I fear for my life," he told them.

***

"Mom, I need your help so much!! I am so scared I can barlie write. Last night Saturday night I come to seggergation for protection from A-unit. The C.O. and staff put me in a cell, C2. Lower. 7. Now just so you know this. The cell mattress smelt like suage like

394

s--- from a tolit."

***

When his mother heard her son's prison sentence a bomb went off in her head. She has teetered on the edge of tears ever since.

How could he survive? Her boy, with his kind heart, who couldn't tolerate as he grew up to be interrupted by the smallest noise in the house when he was tying his shoes?

She would get letters from him every week, like one in which he told her if he died she should do this for his funeral: Play the song "Sweet Child O' Mine," speak with no time limit, serve Dr Pepper and his brother's famous chicken enchiladas.

And another letter with a list of 20 inmates he said had hit, kicked, stomped, teased, threatened and stolen from him. Another list of corrections officers and caseworkers he said lied to him, called him names, provoked him, insulted his mom.

She would clearly hear on a telephone conversation from prison another inmate say to him: *Kill yourself, Austin. Kill yourself.*

It broke her heart that his pleas for relief would be beyond her reach.

***

Austin spent more than four years in prison or jail on

some level of segregation, assessed to be at a high risk of suicide, a moderate risk of violence toward other inmates, and at a high potential to be a victim.

When he threatened suicide, he was stripped down and put on 24-hour watches. He pounded on his cell door and, he said, was locked in five-point restraints, for days, longer than allowed.

He was turned down for parole three times because he didn't get needed programming. They wanted him to go through a substance abuse program, which he tried to do without success.

After the third try, he gave up. "I'm like nah, man, I don't even want your parole cause all you're going to do is keep me on a leash for six months. You're going to watch me, and if I even make one mess up ... you guys will lock me up for it."

He discharged from the hole. And he brought his prison home, the after-effects of withering confinement still felt not just by him, but by his mother and older and younger siblings.

"I live in my own hell, still," he said. "I'll be in one world, but locked up in another in my mind."

***

A loud noise, like the slamming of prison doors, brings Austin back to lockup. Jangling keys means a guard must be outside the door and leads to arguments and outbursts. He doesn't trust. He fears running into prison personnel at the grocery store, church or YMCA.

Ask his mother how it has been since her son left the Lincoln Correctional Center, and there is more than a full minute of silence, her trying to compose herself enough to talk.

"It's been hell, just to see the result of what the guards had done to my son, the institution itself, the system."

The excuse of administrators was that they do their best to train individuals properly, but there are some bad seeds, and they can't weed all of them out, Stinson said.

"But who," she asks, "puts someone in a cage naked on a cement slab and makes them eat and sleep like that when they're suicidal?"

On top of everything else, her second-born son now has severe panic attacks.

She has learned to just listen, and not offer her thoughts.

Saying "I think," reminds him of what he heard in encounters with guards: *I think you'd better shut up. I think you're a piece of s---.*

"If they could only see what they've done to Austin, I think maybe they would rethink how they would treat people," she said.

397

"No they wouldn't, Mom," Austin answers. "They wouldn't care. They wouldn't."

***

Everyone who had contact with Austin recognized he had special needs the prison simply did not have the capacity to address, said Gary Weiss, former Nebraska assistant ombudsman who worked with the family.

His high emotional needs could be wearing on people who did not understand them -- and even those who did.

The state, in general, does not have services for people with special needs who break the law, Weiss said.

It is tempting, if the only tool you have is a hammer, to treat everything as if it were a nail, famed psychologist Abraham Maslow said.

"But that hammer's crushing these folks, just crushing them," Weiss said. "The one-size-fits-all deal that prisons have is just a complete disaster.

Those inmates are going to end up doing some really antisocial things when they get out, he said. It's harmful to public safety.

Two years removed from his job at the Capitol, Weiss sees how dangerous the prison system is for people with disabilities and mental illness. They come out of there not knowing how to get a job, how to raise kids.

"The criminal justice system, the prison system, is destroying communities," he said.

***

For a long time, the prison system did not question the use of long-term segregation, said Nebraska Ombudsman Marshall Lux. They now are starting to do so.

Nebraska's new Corrections director Scott Frakes has made it an issue. While he couldn't address Austin's case specifically, he said, the department continues in its efforts to identify and address specific needs of inmates, and to expand secure mental health housing for inmates at Lincoln Correctional Center.

"The expectation of staff is that the inmate's behavior should not impact the staff member's professionalism," he said.

Nebraska is one of five states selected to get assistance from The Vera Institute of Justice to analyze its use of segregation for inmates, and make recommendations.

Segregation is supposed to isolate inmates who are deemed threats, but Nebraska has increasingly used it to punish inmates, protect the vulnerable or temporarily house those who are awaiting transfer.

399

A law (LB598) passed in this year's legislative session requires the department to come up with new rules and regulations for segregation.

Mentally ill inmates should be in a mental health unit, Lux said. But fewer than 150 mental health beds at the Lincoln Correctional Center aren't enough to handle all those who need them, he said.

***

A tort claim Austin filed with the state, charging emotional, psychological, sexual, physical and spiritual abuse, and asking for $2.1 million for every year he was in isolation, was turned down by the state claims board in June.

It is really hard, he told the board, for a person with autism, to be in isolation and to undergo abuse.

People might say, he understands, that that's what happens when you violate the law.

"But when did it become morally right for a government to be above the law and to be above itself?"

***

Austin decided he could not stay in Nebraska, with all those reminders and without good services.

So with his mother, he found a city on the West Coast, in a state that was friendlier to people with autism and where he could receive respectful rehabilitation. He left Lincoln in late June.

He is getting services there; he feels protected.

But he is still struggling socially, he said. He feels frustrated or aggressive at times, has flashbacks and spends sleepless nights.

"I'm as happy as I can be, and yet still in pain," he said. "I look in my hall closet every time I wake out of sleep to be sure no one is hiding. I look behind my door when I enter my home to be sure I won't be sucker punched."

He never wants to return.

"I would really like to know how Judge Merritt would feel knowing how his decision impacted my son's life and our family's," Stinson said.

The only thing Austin needed was a loving family, which he had, and services that would assist him and protect him from predators, she said. Instead, he was placed in a toxic pool of predators.

"Sending him to prison was the easy way out."

Chapter 41 Closing Chapter

Studies from 2016 show Ten Times more mentally ill people are in jails, and prisons than they are in actual state psychiatric hospitals. This study also showed 356,268 mentally ill people were in prisons, and jails compared to 35,000 mentally ill people in psychiatric hospitals.

I was born in Southern California, and I was raised in the mountains. During my birth there were complications that took place. My mother's womb came open before my birth. During that process, my mother lost a lot of water. The fact that there was a hole in my mother's amniotic sac was crucial. I had no water, and the doctors had very little faith. The doctors said I would most likely be a still birth. My mother and father didn't like that news. Story has it that my father prayed all night and cried all night. The next day as my father laid near my mother's bedside, the doctors did an evaluation, and the hole had healed. The doctors said I might have a chance. Story has it my mother gave birth to me soon after. I was six weeks mature, and I had an odd birth. My birth was a dry birth, and there wasn't any liquid to help my mother deliver me. The doctor looked me over and evaluated me. He explained to my parents that there was no sign of physical abnormality.

However, that didn't mean there wouldn't be any neurological abnormalities.

From that day on, as a child I had many autistic tendencies. I didn't socialize with others, and I kept everything in order. My toys and my books would all have to be in order. I even took cleaning supplies, and I cleaned my toys with a wash rag. I would wash my hands multiple times a day, and my behavior was often questioned. I lived in Southern California until I was about five years old. Story has it moving was my father's idea, and my mother wanted to stay in California. My father, however, wanted to move us to Nebraska. So we did, and we traveled about three days in a beat up station wagon. During the drive Blind Melon was on the radio. My brothers and I listened to the song "No More Rain" on our way to Nebraska. We would sleep in the car during the night, and we would drive during the day. Once we arrived, we moved into a trailer park, and I hated it. It was no longer the West Coast, and dreams were no longer reachable. My family and I lived in Lincoln, Nebraska. I went to an elementary school called West Lincoln Elementary. During class my teacher would lock me in the classroom closet. She would keep me in the closet the entire day. I reported the abuse to my mother, and I was transferred schools that year. I attended Belmont Elementary, and needless to say it was the same. I was bullied by children and teachers during class. I was hated and teased every day. The teachers allowed other students to bully me. I was very overwhelmed by home life and school life. As a child I often threatened to commit suicide. I did this in fear of my surroundings, even though I wasn't truly suicidal. It was a form of attention seeking. I took a knife and held the knife to my throat. I did this while I was with my home counselor. She was so stupid that she thought I was displaying poor behavior, when in fact I was seeking attention. I wanted to be noticed, and I wanted the abuse to stop. The abuse from my father and the abuse from the school.

While living in Nebraska I was often in the children's psychiatric hospital. Testing would be done by doctors and so-called professionals. However, in Nebraska autism was not well known. Autism to a Nebraska psychiatric doctor had a smaller window for approval. I had five to six different doctors during my childhood. Unfortunately, because autism was such a difficult disorder to understand, I was miss-diagnosed while growing up in the early nineteen nineties.

I missed California, and I always hoped that my father would move us back. That hope was only a hope, and it never came to pass. My father was a difficult man to be around. He drank alcohol every day, and he abused me quite often. He would slap me, and drag me, and even throw me against our basement wall. He was a correctional officer in the nineteen nineties, and he worked his way up to be a counselor for the Nebraska Department of Corrections. He earned his masters degree in psychology, and no one knew the real Jeff Bower like I did. My father was a drunk, and he displayed his anger only at home. He was two different people. The best way to describe him would be Dr. Jekyll and Mr. Hyde. He would act well managed in society and at work. Then he would come home, and he would beat on me and my mother.

The process of working with the psychiatric doctors was a failure, mainly because they were not educated enough about autism to say bluntly that I had autism. Instead they diagnosed me with obsessive compulsive disorder, mood disorder, and Tourette's syndrome, which today Tourette's is acknowledged to be on the spectrum of autism.

My father was diagnosed with stage three lung cancer when I was seventeen years old. He smoked on a regular basis. I guess he thought smoking would never kill him. Well, he thought wrong. He struggled with cancer for about a full year, and there was nothing the doctors could do for him. I was eighteen and still in high school when my father kicked the bucket. He died of cancer on January 12th, 2007. As a family we were torn apart and in dire need of healing. My mother had a very challenging time throughout the grieving process. In fact, she wasn't sure how to help me.

As I aged in the system and worked with psychiatric doctors throughout my life, not one of them diagnosed me with autism. My mother filed an application for me to receive developmental disability services in Nebraska, which of course they denied me for services. I was lost with no hope, and I didn't know how to care for myself. While living in Lincoln I picked up some bad habits, such as smoking and drinking. I hung around dangerous people, and most of the time I didn't know what I was getting myself into. My mother wouldn't allow me to live with her because of my special needs. She was grieving the death of her spouse, and she couldn't take care of me. So my mother sent me to a group home, and I was given a lack of services. I was forced to move out of the group home because the staff didn't like me. I soon became homeless, and I lived on the streets. I slept in basements to apartment complexes and old worn out building. I was still in high school during all of this. Believe it or not, I graduated high school. I received my diploma from Lincoln Southeast High School in 2009.

About two months later I met Hawkboy. I didn't know Hawkboy's background, and I didn't know he was a felon. I only knew what he told me, and he told me lies. Because of the robbery, I spent some of the most important years of my life in prison.

My mother and I filed a tort claim through risk management. The tort claim was for 2.2 million dollars for each year I spent in isolation. The tort claim was written by me. My mother had documentation from the prison. In the documentation there were many statements made by employees of the state. Some of the employees said I was at risk and vulnerable to suicide. Other employees said I was prone to the vulnerability of other inmates. The employees of the department of corrections even stated I was safer in solitary confinement. My tort claim was picked up by a civil rights attorney.

After serving my sentence in Nebraska, I moved to Oregon. While living in Eugene, Oregon I had an evaluation completed by a doctor, Jack Martin. My mother was requested to send the documentation she had to the division of Lane County Developmental Disability Services. My mother faxed all of the information to the division of Lane County. After the evaluation I qualified for developmental disability services, which raises a larger question of why Nebraska denied me. I lived in an adult foster home for five months. During my stay in the adult foster home, I attempted suicide. I swallowed over one hundred pills. I was placed in the McKenzie Willamette Medical Center for two days, which is in Springfield, Oregon. While living in my AFH home, I received wrap around services. The foster care providers cooked, cleaned, and transported me to my appointments and outings, meeting all my basic needs. My foster care providers also drove me to the food mart. They would allow me to help pick out meals.

Lane County consisted of Springfield, OR. and Eugene, OR., and I lived in both cities. It was a beautiful place to live in. However, I moved back to Nebraska because I wasn't close to family. I needed to be near my mother and siblings.

Due to my post traumatic stress disorder, upon my return to Nebraska, I was placed into a psychiatric hospital. I underwent many evaluations, and I was placed on various medications. I had many physical altercations with hospital employees and patients. I was often placed into full bed restraints, and I was often placed in isolation. The state hospital was a horrible experience. The employees were childish, and the patients were mentally sick. I was housed in building five of the Lincoln Regional Center. I spent one year inside those walls for intense psychological treatment. During my stay in the Lincoln Regional Center, my mother became my legal guardian.

Upon my release my mother applied for me to receive, developmental disability services. This was the second time we applied in Nebraska. This time I had three different doctors, who previously diagnosed me with autism, and I also had paperwork from Oregon. My mother received more documentation while being my legal guardian. Even with all of that, developmental disability services of Nebraska denied me again. The injustice was unending, and even with the federal regulations for me, and not against me, the state of Nebraska still chose to be sinister. My mother is still attempting to win this battle, but Nebraska is not making it easy.

I currently live with my brother, and he helps me with day to day life. Someday I hope to receive developmental disability services in Nebraska. It has been an ongoing battle, but I hope something happens soon. Life has been a challenge, and I haven't given up on hope. I hope my story inspires other stories like mine to come forward. I pray that one day the system will be forever changed, so individuals like me don't have to suffer. I wish my book had a happier ending. My lawsuit never went to court, and I was never given a settlement. However, I was given records and documentation from my court hearings and prison experience. I also have two newspaper articles supporting my written work. So I chose to write a book after everything I went through. Writing this story was not easy, but it's my only way to receive justice.

Made in the USA
Middletown, DE
24 September 2023